COPING WITH STAMMERING
A SELF-HELP APPROACH

TRUDY STEWART & JACKIE TURNBULL are experienced speech and language therapists based in Leeds. They specialize in working with adults and children who stammer. They have written articles and books for professionals and a self-help book for parents of children who stammer.

They are actively involved in the British Stammering Association and in generally promoting the needs of those who stammer in the workplace and in society as a whole.

They believe the best outcomes are achieved when they work in partnership with their clients, families and others. They see each person who stammers as an individual and tailor their therapy to individual needs.

Overcoming Common Problems Series

For a full list of titles please contact
Sheldon Press, Marylebone Road, London NW1 4DU

Overcoming Common Problems

Coping with Stammering
A self-help approach

Trudy Stewart
and
Jackie Turnbull

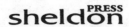

First published in Great Britain in 1997 by
Sheldon Press, SPCK, Marylebone Road, London NW1 4DU

© Trudy Stewart and Jackie Turnbull 1997

British Library Cataloguing-in-Publication Data
A catalogue record for this book is available from the British Library

ISBN 0–85969–758–4

Photoset by Deltatype Limited, Birkenhead, Merseyside
Printed in Great Britain by
Biddles Ltd, Guildford and King's Lynn

Contents

Throughout the book people who stammer have been referred to as 'they', and in some instances 'clients', this has been used for clarity. We would like our readers to note that we do not believe there is a collective noun for people who stammer; each person is an individual, with difficulties peculiar to him or her. We hope that our work with individuals reflects this view.

Dedication

To all those adults we have met in our clinics. They have taught us to view each person who stammers as an individual with a unique past, present and future.

To our families who still love us, despite our constant cries of 'I'll be with you in a minute, I'm just finishing this chapter'.

Acknowledgements

We would like to thank all our clients, past and present, for sharing their experiences with us and helping us learn about stammering. In particular, we are grateful to Mark Birdsall, Diane Buckle, Daniel Hunter, Andrew Johnstone, Nasser Karimi, Maria Neary, Mike Peace, Peter Smith and Bryan Wood for their special, personal contributions.

We also acknowledge the assistance that Rita Greer, speech and language therapist and hypnotherapist, and Stewart T. Lightbody, Director of the Halifax Clinic of Natural Medicine, gave us when writing some of the sections about alternative therapies.

Introduction

When writing a book such as this, the aim of which is to help other people, we need to assume we know something about our readers. Certainly we have met lots of people who stammer and have worked for many years in the area, so we do know quite a bit about stammering. One crucial thing that we have learnt is that no one individual who stammers is like another. There will be some important similarities – perhaps in the way the person stammers, the way they react to their stammer or, alternatively, the effect it has had on their life – but there will be many differences too. Because of this it is vital that we respond to those who stammer as individuals and not assume that they are all the same.

In writing this book we accept that we are unable to cater for each individual reader's concerns. However, we will aim to cover as many possibilities and eventualities as we can and ask that you consider those that apply to you, or to those you know who stammer, and skim over issues which do not apply.

Given that stammering is such an individual problem, you might feel that we are foolish to try to offer suggestions of a general nature to help people cope with it. You may be right! However, we decided we had to attempt it as many of our clients and their partners and friends asked us to recommend literature on stammering, and there seemed very little available which suited their needs. Some requested background reading as they started a course of therapy or for their partners and/or family members. Many, although stammering themselves, knew very little about the theories of stammering, how it develops, what maintains it and so on, and wanted to know more. Others wanted some information on the different types of therapy available before deciding which one was appropriate for them. Finally, we had some clients who were approaching the end of a programme of therapy and needed a book to remind them of techniques they had learnt and specific strategies to help them maintain those skills. We have considered all these issues, and include sections on background information on stammering, what it is and how it develops, how a person might approach changing their stammer, the different types of therapy available and a lot of ideas on techniques and maintenance strategies. We have also included details of some techniques which can be difficult to learn on your own. In such cases, we make it clear that it may be best to seek professional help.

Throughout the book you will find examples of the personal experiences

1

of those who stammer. You may well find that these accounts are the most useful parts of the book. This fits very well with our belief that while we, as speech and language therapists, have some knowledge and information which facilitates change, the real source of practical help is the experience of each person who stammers. Individuals who stammer are the *real* experts on stammering, and we readily acknowledge that much of this book is based on what we have learnt from our clients.

1
What is stammering?

First of all, stammering is the same as stuttering. The only difference is that the term stuttering is more commonly used in America and Canada. Stammering is the word used in Britain and the one we will use throughout the book, but its meaning is identical to that of stuttering.

Most people are able to identify when a person is stammering severely. People may not be able to tell you exactly what happens when a person stammers, but they can tell the difference between someone who does not stammer and a person who stammers most of the time. In actual fact, there is a fine line dividing fluency and stammering, and for every listener that dividing line will be different; we all have distinct 'tolerance levels'. It is interesting to consider that fact for a moment, think about it from a listener's perspective and note how this makes stammering quite unlike a number of other speech problems. For example, as a listener you are usually aware when a child or an adult is unable to say an 'r' sound. Generally this difficulty is present in all aspects of their speech – when they read, talk to a variety of people and when they sing. It will also be noticeable to any other listener present in the room. Stammering, though, is a whole different ball game! First, it can vary so much that it is only perceived in certain situations – perhaps when the person talks on the phone, but not when they talk to their young child and certainly never when they sing in the bath. Second, some listeners may not be aware of it at all, while others are much more tuned in to it. This may be because they notice speech generally or perhaps they have heard a person who stammers before – they may be married to one! Having said that, there is much more of an 'interactive' element to stammering than any other speech problem, in that a person who stammers can be affected by other people and by the situation in which the words are spoken. This aspect of stammering is peculiar to it, and something which makes it difficult to treat and, as many of our clients would agree, difficult to live with.

What exactly is stammering? If we can be technical for a moment, stammering is usually defined as a communication disorder which affects the flow and timing of speech. Thus, a person is able to formulate what they wish to say, they know the words which will convey their meaning and they can construct a sentence which obeys the grammatical rules of language – all without difficulty. The problem arises sometimes when they try to move the muscles of their larynx (or voice box), lips, tongue, palate, jaw and so on to articulate the sounds of the words. At this point the process breaks down, even though there appears to be nothing physically wrong with the person's mouth or other parts associated with speech. However, when they begin to talk in certain situations, their muscles or the movements themselves do not appear to be co-ordinated – the muscles can go into spasm or lock and the speaker is unable to make the sound they wish to. They try to push the sound out by increasing the muscle tension, they stop, take in a bigger breath and have another run at it, perhaps changing the word to one they are likely to have more success with, or maybe they give up and stop speaking altogether. At the end of it all they feel angry, frustrated, isolated from others who seem to have no difficulty communicating, and it saps their energy, confidence levels and self-esteem.

Looking for answers

The state of the art

There are reports of stammering as far back as 2,500 years ago. It is mentioned in 20th-century BC hieroglyphics, in the Bible and in the Koran. There is ample documentary evidence on the treatment of stammering from the 16th century onwards, but none of it could be recommended today. Early medics would remove pieces of the tongue, insert hot needles into the mouth or secure the jaw and tongue with metal strapping.

Yet, despite this long history and attempts over hundreds of years to alleviate stammering, we still do not have a cure. However, we are making progress. We know some of the things that contribute to the development of stammering in children and factors which maintain and sustain it into adulthood. In fact, speech and language therapists who specialize in this field are reporting good results in preventing its further development beyond childhood. This is good news for future generations, but the picture is not quite as rosy for adults who are stammering now. Having said that, we would urge you not to give up hope! We continue to improve our therapeutic skills and have a number of techniques which can give some relief and help those who stammer live a fulfilling life.

We both can tell you about clients who have benefited from help, but one in particular springs to mind.

Richard's story

Richard came from a family in which his stammer was never discussed. It was accepted that Richard stammered and that, essentially, was the end of it. However, he suffered severe teasing in school and his schooldays were a living nightmare with no one to talk to about it.

In later life, he had a road traffic accident at a time when he thought things were getting better. He lost his job prospects, a long-standing relationship and his hope. He asked for therapy for his stammer shortly after this and described how he felt his life was at a low ebb and how he had had just about enough. He had one year of therapy and did very well. Through hard work and a lot of risk taking, he achieved some good control over his speech and regained his self-respect. We heard him on the radio recently promoting self-help groups for those who stammer in his area and proving to himself and everyone who heard him that there is life with a stammer.

Causes: fact or fiction?

Over the years, a number of theories about stammering, what causes it and so on, have developed. From our own experience we have been aware that friends, other professionals and clients themselves hold certain beliefs about why people stammer which are not based on evidence but more on myth. In this section we will examine a range of these theories and sort out the facts from the fiction.

The nervous personality: fact or fiction?

Perhaps the most common myth we have encountered is that stammering is a result of the person being of an anxious disposition. Thus, stammering is seen as an outward manifestation of anxiety when speaking in a particular situation. It is quite clear how this belief may have arisen. Many fluent speakers become less fluent, more hesitant and even display stammering-type speech when they are nervous. We ourselves can recall numerous occasions when we have given important presentations and found that the anxiety we have felt has disrupted the flow of our speech, at least for the initial few minutes. Thus, many people who do not stammer assume that the stammering they hear is the same hesitancy that they themselves experience when they are nervous, and generalize from this experience to ascribe this as the cause of the non-fluent person's difficulty.

The problem with this belief is that while the speech *sounds* nervous, the person stammering is no more or less nervous than anyone else. From our experience, we would describe few of our clients as nervous. Many of them are highly articulate, erudite speakers – only their stammering makes them appear differently. Someone who stammers can feel nervous because they anticipate stammering in a particular context, but this does not make them a 'nervous' or 'anxious' person. This view is further supported by research which shows that people who stammer are no less confident, no more anxious or nervous than anyone else in the general population.

Stammering as a result of trauma: fact or fiction?

Many of our clients can recall significant traumatic events which they associate with the beginning of their stammering. Ones that spring to mind include a tonsillectomy, a gorilla at the zoo, a period of separation from a parent and a change of schools or move to a different location.

There are a number of ways of looking at this:

- The event was not significant in itself, but the timing was. By this we mean that it occurred at a time when other important things were happening in the child's life. This particular event may only have been significant in terms of tipping an already tilting scale in favour of non-fluent speech.
- The event may not have been significant but somehow the child's perception was aroused and they became more acutely aware that all was not well with their speech.
- The event was significant and did contribute to the development of non-fluent speech in the child. There is certainly some evidence that traumatic events can give rise to stammering in adulthood. If the event results in some damage to the central nervous system, then a person can acquire stammering speech. On the other hand, a traumatic shock, such as witnessing a violent event, and a build-up of severe anxiety over either a short or extended period have reportedly resulted in people acquiring stammers in adulthood. Many of these latter examples can be seen as a psychological response to what has happened and, indeed, they do appear to resolve themselves if appropriate support and counselling are given. This is in contrast to the stammers which have a neurological origin.

Infectious stammering: fact or fiction?

Some clients have reported that they began stammering when they sat next to a child in class who stammered. Other concerns have been expressed by parents who worry that their child might 'catch' a stammer from either another child or from the other parent in the family who stammers.

We can categorically state that stammering is not infectious in this way. In order for it to be transmitted like this, from child to child, a micro-organism of some kind, such as a virus or bacteria, would need to be involved, and no such organism has been identified.

However, with regard to transmission in families, there is some evidence that stammering has a genetic link. This is a very complicated area and the research to date is confusing to say the least. Let us summarize the more definitive studies so far:

- The incidence of stammering among relatives of people who stammer is 14 per cent, whereas in the general population the figure is only 1 per cent.
- If someone in your family stammers, you are three times more likely to stammer yourself than if you had been born into a family in which no one stammered.
- The severity of the stammer is not an important determining factor, so if Uncle Clive has a severe stammer you are no more likely to inherit it than if he stammered only mildly.
- If a female member of your family stammers, there is a greater chance of you inheriting a stammer yourself.
- If you are female, there is more chance of you recovering.

Stammering can be learnt: fact or fiction?

As a behaviour, stammering can be learnt in the same way that you could learn how to speak with a Geordie or a Cockney accent. Some people could do it quite easily and others would struggle to perfect it. They would need to speak in that way for a good many months, even years perhaps, for them to feel as if it was their normal speaking voice. The question that springs to mind is why would they wish to do this? If they were actors, you could understand their wishing to master a particular tone of voice or manner of address – it adds to the characterization and, ultimately, the performance. However, why someone should choose to learn stammering is something we do not readily comprehend.

Parents cause stammering: fact or fiction?

Parents do not cause stammering.

About 50 years ago, a speech and language pathologist in America called Wendel Johnson devised and wrote a theory on the development of stammering in children. His theory laid the responsibility squarely on the parents' or carers' shoulders. He argued that because they labelled the child's early stumblings over words as stammering, the child then grew up to think of their speech in that way, too.

We now know that this theory was simplistic and that the reality is much more complicated. Children may well be influenced by how their parents perceive them, but they will also be influenced by many other factors, such as their own beliefs, their peer group and so on.

More recently, a number of other factors have also been identified as contributing to the development of non-fluent speech. These include:

- the child's ability to control their muscles;
- their rhythmical skills;
- how much speech is demanded of them in certain situations;
- how quickly other people speak to them;
- whether or not they are allowed to complete their turn to speak before someone else jumps in.

This is quite a long list. As far as the role of parents goes in all this, it is clear that the responsibility does not rest solely on their shoulders. Instead, there are likely to be a number of factors, which only become significant when they occur together.

Stammering is caused by a physical defect: fact or fiction?

First, we can definitely state that stammering is not caused by a defect in the structure of the tongue, lips, roof of the mouth or throat. Large tongues, short tongues, tongue ties and so on do not feature in the majority of people who stammer. These structures – the muscles contained in them and the nerve supply to them – are the same as those of a fluent speaker. Having said that, there is some evidence to suggest that some people who stammer differ from those who do not in a number of other ways:

- the time it takes to start the vocal chords vibrating in the voice box;
- the way speech is processed in the brain;
- brain wave patterns during speech;
- blood flow differences in the brain during speech.

However, having read the literature, there are many conflicting reports and it is clear that no one is sure enough to say stammering is caused by X. We think the jury is still out!

Stammering is caused by being forced to use the non-preferred hand for writing: fact or fiction?

There was a theory popular in the 1930s which proposed that stammering was caused by ambiguous or confused 'lateral dominance'. By the 1940s, this theory was largely disproved and fell out of favour. However, in more recent times, as we have noted above, differences in which hemisphere of the brain processes sound and the brain wave patterns of the two sides have been noted in some people who stammer. This is likely to be an area of continued research.

8

Stammering can be affected by eating certain foods: fact or fiction?

Stammering can be found in almost every culture in the world. As we encounter people who stammer from cultures other than our own, we have become aware that there are different beliefs about the origins of stammering. In some cultures, there are beliefs that stammering may be caused by eating or drinking certain things. Sometimes the temperature appears to be an important element in this belief (such as with ice-cream), while on other occasions it is linked to specific products (like cola drinks).

For this to be valid, stammering would have to be associated with diet, nutrition or the metabolic system in some way. No evidence has been found to suggest that this is the case.

People who stammer are different from the 'average': fact or fiction?

Approximately 1 per cent of the population stammer. This rises to about 5 per cent if you ask who has stammered at some point in their life. That is quite a lot of people.

Interestingly, if you stammer, you are more likely to be male than female as the ratio of males to females who stammer is estimated to be around 5 to 1. While there may be a genetic link of some kind in a number of these cases, there is very little else that is common to them all. In fact, they are as different from each other as one would expect a large slice of the general population to be.

Stammering can affect anyone – you do not have to be intelligent, sporty, artistic, middle class or vote a particular way to be eligible! There is certainly no evidence to suggest that those who stammer are any less intelligent, less able than anyone else. They just talk in a different way.

What do we know about stammering?

How many people stammer?

As mentioned above, about 1 per cent of the population report they stammer, with more males than females across the older age ranges. There is some research which shows that this ratio changes with age. In younger children, there are slightly more females than males who stammer, making the figures more like 2 or 3 to 1. However, as this figure changes when you look at the incidence in adults, it seems likely that there is a greater chance of females recovering than males.

Interestingly, many famous people have stammered, including Winston Churchill, Marilyn Monroe, King George VI and Rowan Atkinson. This appears to underline the fact that stammering is something which can affect any type of person and does not have to stop you doing what you want to with your life.

When does stammering start?

It usually starts in childhood, and we will discuss this in a later chapter. It can also be acquired at a later date, but this is less usual.

The variability of stammering

Stammering is unpredictable. Someone who stammers will often report that it appears to have a life and a will of its own. Of course it does not, but its variability can frequently make it seem so. It can vary in the space of a day, depending on the pressure felt in a situation, how relaxed, how tired they are or how long it takes them to get going in the morning. More often, people tell us about its cyclical nature, how you can have a good spell of a few days, perhaps even a week or two, and then it all seems to fall apart again.

Not only does it vary within an individual, it varies tremendously from person to person. No one's stammer is like another's. Because of this, we ask our clients to use 'I' when talking about stammering, rather than 'we'. (It also helps the client own their thoughts and feelings.) There are similarities of course, but it is wrong to make the assumption that feelings, emotions, behaviour or symptoms are the same for all those who stammer.

Phenomena associated with stammering

Although stammering is very individual, a number of phenomena are shared by many people who stammer. These have been identified over several decades of research.

- *Novelty* If a person who stammers is asked to talk in a slightly different way to how they normally talk, the resulting speech is usually more fluent, at least for a while. This new way of talking can take the form of a different voice (of a higher or lower pitch, an increase or decrease in volume, whispering and speaking at a different speed). One well-documented account is of Desmosthenes, a classical Greek scholar, who achieved fluency by putting small pebbles in his mouth (not a tactic we would recommend!). However, this is, in fact, a novelty effect. Once the novelty has worn off, the speech will return to the original fluency level. You may have experienced this effect yourself if you stammer. Perhaps during a long or difficult stammer you tried something new to enable you to get the sound out. You maybe hit your thigh, nodded your head or tapped your foot and, amazingly, it worked. 'Great,' you thought, 'I've cracked this now. I'll do that every time I get stuck and I won't have any problems.' Unfortunately, as we have seen, it works for a while and then does not make any difference. The only problem is that the thigh slapping, head nodding or foot tapping becomes part of your stammering behaviour.

- *Talking to yourself when you are alone or speaking to children or animals* Many people who stammer report that their speech is much better, if not fluent, when they talk to themselves, young children or a family pet. In a discussion with a female client this phenomenon was raised. It was her belief that this occurred because these were speaking situations in which she experienced no pressure. Her listeners had no preconceptions about her or her speech. She did not have to try to be fluent or, indeed, try to be anything other than herself. We really do not know why speech is better in these situations, but this seems as good an explanation as any we might think of and fits in with a number of modern theories on stammering.

- *Singing* It is an accepted fact that stammering does not usually occur when you are singing. Certainly we have only met one or two people who have claimed otherwise. (However, knowing stammering as we do, we have not ruled out the possibility of meeting more exceptions to this particular rule!) This phenomenon has been used in the past in various therapy techniques. A person would be encouraged to use an exaggerated intonation pattern, almost a sing-song sort of voice, or, in some cases, told to 'sing it' when they could not say it. This is not used nowadays. It is such a bizarre way of talking that arguably it is preferable to stammer. As to why it should be that singing eliminates stammering, there is no definite answer. However, the best guess we can currently make is that the exaggerated rhythmical pattern involved in singing helps you predict how the sentence or phrase will proceed. The melody lays down a template, if you like, which the speaker or singer only has to follow. This takes some of the effort out of speaking and perhaps makes it an easier process.

- *Reading along with or immediately after another person* It has been observed that when a person who stammers is required to read a passage at the same time as another fluent speaker, then they are likely to stammer less. Similarly, if they are asked to read, this time speaking the same words directly after the other person, the effect will be the same (this is known as *shadowing*). It is unclear why this happens. It may be related to the ability of the person who stammers to process what they hear. In some way, hearing another person read alongside them as they speak the same words corrects the feedback they receive. Another theory is that, as with singing, a new template is established which makes it easier for the non-fluent person to speak.

- *Adaptation* This technical term refers to a frequently recorded phenomenon relating once again to reading. In this instance, the person who stammers is asked to read the same passage a number of times (usually

11

three). On each occasion the number of stammers and the places where the stammers occurred in the passage are recorded. What has been found is that the stammering decreases significantly during the course of the three readings. If, however, the exercise is prolonged over further readings, then the effect is lost. This has implications for people who stammer. The inference seems to be that it is worth practising your speech to a certain degree, but you can overdo it and lose any possible benefit.

- *Adjacency* Another technical term. Unfortunately, it refers to a phenomenon that is of questionable benefit. In this instance, those who stammer are asked to read a passage. The positions of the stammers are marked on the passage and the stammered words removed. It has been found that when the passage is re-read, without the stammered words, stammering then occurs on the words adjacent to the original stammered words. Now why should that be? Perhaps people remember where they stammered and therefore expect to stammer in the same places? Maybe it is related to breathing or the position in the sentence? Any answers to this puzzle would be gratefully received!

Other factors associated with fluency

Pressure

Most of our clients say that their speech is at its worst when they feel under pressure. This can include times when they need to say specific words, like giving their name and address, saying a technical term for which there is no alternative or answering the phone at work in the required way, stating the department and a friendly greeting. (Of course, once the word has been said by someone else it can often be said without a stammer at all, which is frustrating to say the least!)

Fluency often deteriorates in situations which put speech under pressure. Once again the telephone springs to mind. Here all the onus is on the speaking voice – there are no facial expressions, gestures or other non-verbal cues to help the communication. The speech is all there is to convey the message. No wonder it is a nightmare for those with speech problems.

Other situations frequently mentioned include interviews, the marriage ceremony, giving talks to groups of people and other public speaking situations. Interestingly, these are also occasions when people who do *not* stammer feel anxious and uncomfortable.

Physical factors

It has long been recognized that stammering can get worse when a person is physically below par. If you are ill, emotionally upset or just at the end of a long, hard day, then the chances are that your speech will reflect your physical state. For a fluent speaker, this may show up as an inability to think of the right words to say or getting sounds in words muddled, like tefelone or hang coater. For a person who stammers, it is more likely to be realized as more stammering.

On the other hand, the level of relaxation a person can achieve usually works in favour of fluency. The more relaxed you are in a speaking situation, the greater the chance of improved fluency. In therapy, some professionals recommend practising attaining a relaxed state for this reason. However, it is important that you are able to achieve this muscular state in a speaking situation and not just practise it in isolation (this is discussed further in a later chapter).

You can become relaxed in other ways, including by means of hypnosis, the intake of alcohol and some drugs. We will discuss hypnosis and other alternative forms of medicine later in the book. However, it should be noted that, for some, imbibing substances, such as alcohol, can have a less predictable effect on fluency and, of course, can be harmful in the long term. For example, a number of our clients report that their speech is actually worse after they have had a pint or two (their reports after greater amounts are less reliable!) Others say that their speech is better after small amounts and then deteriorates as they drink more. It is obviously an individual issue, but not one we would recommend as a viable option over a prolonged period of time.

Linguistic factors

A lot of research was carried out in the 1930s and 1940s to establish whether or not there were things about the way language is spoken – for example, the sounds used or the structure of sentences – which contributed to stammering. The results are widely accepted these days and can be summarized as follows:

- Stammers are more likely to occur on consonants than vowels.
- No one consonant makes people stammer more than any other.
- Stammering occurs more often when people start to speak than when they have been speaking for a little while.
- Stammering occurs more often on words which carry the information in a sentence, the nouns and verbs rather than the articles 'the' or 'a'.
- Stammering occurs more frequently with longer words that have several syllables.

Is there a cure?

The short answer is 'no', there is no cure for stammering in adults. However, after several decades of trying to alleviate stammering in both children and adults, some success has been achieved. Certainly it would appear from

13

research that the incidence in late childhood is decreasing. This suggests that we are getting better at treating childhood non-fluency.

With respect to adults, we continue to try and develop techniques which will bring about a significant and long-lasting change. The problem has been the 'long-lasting' bit. It has proved comparatively easy to help a person who stammers to change their way of speaking in a short time. However, our experience (and that of other professionals) is that this change can be short-lived, the person soon returning to the clinic requesting further help.

However, we personally have learnt much from others working with different clients and in different settings. Individually we have pursued different paths, including studying abroad, working with counsellors and family therapists, researching into different areas of stammering and experimenting with different therapy options. In our professional collaboration, all of these experiences have been shared and used in some way to improve our practice. We now feel confident that we have a range of therapy strategies that will enable someone to make the changes they wish to make and develop their own 'toolbox' with which they can maintain these changes in the long term. These ideas will form the basis of Chapter 10, but we would recommend that you read the intervening chapters first!

Summary

In this chapter we have painted a picture of what stammering is and how individual it can be. We have tried to dispel some of the myths associated with the problem and have given you some of the more concrete facts about stammering, based on research findings to date. We are aware that the information we have on stammering is constantly developing and changing and we, as practising clinicians, have to keep pace with this. We are conscious, too, that as a result, the material in this chapter may become out of date and be added to from time to time. We would therefore encourage you to keep a beady eye on some of the scientific journals listed at the end of the Further reading section at the back of the book if you wish to know about the latest developments.

2

Getting to know a stammer

If you have a stammer, you may look at the title of this chapter and think you do not need to read this section, that your personal experience is such that, really, you know all there is to know. You may well be right. Perhaps you do have a very good working knowledge of what exactly happens when you stammer. However, there will be some of you who do not stammer yourselves and need a greater understanding of the problem that someone close to you is going through. There may also be some of you who do stammer, yet, despite your personal experience of it, have not analysed objectively what goes on during a stammering event. Let's face it, stammering is not the most pleasant condition ever experienced and it would be very natural to try and forget it or put it to the back of your mind as soon as it was over.

All this agreed, it is also important to remember that if you want to change something, you must know precisely what it is you are going to change. Like an athlete who wishes to improve their style in order to improve their time or perform better in some other way, every muscle movement is analysed to the nth degree. This is done in order to eliminate the factors that are impairing their effectiveness, and they will then work on developing those aspects that enhance their performance. So it is with speech. In order to improve your fluency and decrease the impact stammering has on your communication, you must get to know your stammer inside out, understand the factors that precipitate it, how it starts, which muscles are involved at the beginning, how it feels, how the stammer progresses, what brings the stammer to a close and how you feel once it is finished.

That seems like an enormous list to cope with all at once, and so it is. In order to make this process more manageable, it is useful to break stammering down into a number of 'bite-size' pieces. This is the process therapists use to help them understand what is going on when they analyse any adult's stammer.

Analysing your stammer

Stammering can be divided into two parts.

- The *outward* signs, the things that other people can see and hear you do when you are trying to get your words or sounds out (this is known as the *overt stammer*).

- The *inward or internal* aspects of stammering, which are the aspects of stammering that are not so obvious to your listeners. They may be little tricks or strategies you have developed to hide your stammering, like avoiding certain words or sounds that you know you will stammer on, or feelings you have when you stammer (this is known as the *covert stammer*).

The outward signs

Let us consider these signs in some detail. In some ways they can be the easiest to identify, but may be most distressing to those who have stammers which are very obvious. Which of the following do you do?

Repetitions

Some people have a type of stammer which involves saying particular speech units over and over again. These units may be sounds (as in 'ssssounds'), syllables or parts of words ('re re re repetitions') and/or words. It is less usual for longer units to be repeated in the stammering of adults, although some people who stammer will repeat phrases or parts of sentences as a run-in to a word or sound they find difficult to say. More of this later. (In addition, some people who do not stammer may repeat these longer units – this can be one of the aspects that differentiates more fluent speakers.)

The way these repetitions are said is also worth looking at. They may occur in an easy fashion or be said with lots of tension in the speech muscles and sound as if they are forced or pushed out. In addition, the speed of the repetitions should be noted. Are they spoken in a slow way or are they hurried and produced in rapid bursts which feel out of control?

Finally, consider how long the repetitions last on average – a second or two, several seconds or longer? It can be worth carrying out a small experiment to find this out. The likelihood is that it *feels* longer to you than it actually is – a bit like when you are waiting for something to happen, for the kettle to boil or a bus to arrive! You should try to observe, and ideally time, how long your repetitions last on a number of occasions, in a variety of situations. It may be that the repetitions will appear different when you are under pressure, feel more anxious or perhaps when you are speaking to different people.

Prolongations and/or blocks

Some people have a stammer in which they hold on to a particular sound for longer than seems appropriate. This holding, as we could call it, can involve making sound or may be silent. So, for example, a person who is having difficulty with the 'l' of the word 'lie' will usually have an associated audible sound. Their mouth will be open, their tongue tip touching the roof of their mouth, approximately in the middle, and their vocal chords vibrating to make the noise we identify with the 'l' sound. On the other hand, a person can be trying to say the word 'pie' and get stuck on the first sound. Their lips will be placed tightly together for the 'p', but there will be no noise. This type of stammer, in which there is no sound, is more commonly known as a *block*.

If this is part of your stammering, then it is worth considering the following:

- First, are there any sounds in particular that you get stuck on – for example, does it tend to be consonants rather than vowels and, if so, which ones?
- You should also think about where the 'block' or the 'holding' is located – for example, in the illustrations we gave above the person tried to say 'pie' and the 'p' was stuck in their mouth, at the point where their lips met to make the 'p' sound (there may also have been some tension in the voice box or larynx which prevented air from moving through their vocal chords).
- Next, think about how long the prolonged sound or block generally lasts – an average number of seconds is adequate for this purpose.
- Finally, consider when this type of stammering occurs in your speech – when you are more relaxed, or more tense, at the end of the day or the beginning – and listing some of the situations or occasions you notice them can be helpful as you can then look for any pattern at a later date.

'Added extras' when talking

Another aspect of stammering is the extra sounds or words which are added in, perhaps without consciously thinking or maybe as a deliberate attempt to give the speaker more time or help them get started. Consider these examples and see which apply to your speech:

- extra sounds before certain words or sounds on which you anticipate problems, such as 'nn Jackie', 'll Trudy';
- adding sounds (say, 'mmm hello'), words (such as 'actually') or phrases (for example, 'you know');
- using other sounds when talking, such as coughing, clearing your throat and sniffing;
- using 'ums' and 'ers' a lot of the time.

Breathing

For several decades, people have noticed that many of those who stammer also have breathing problems. However, what is not clear is whether the breathing is the 'chicken' or the 'egg', that is, whether the difficulties with

17

normal breathing patterns are a result of the stammer or whether they themselves precipitate the stammer in some way.

The want of an answer to this question has not prevented therapists and others from working on breathing when attempting to eliminate or control stammering. Undoubtedly, for some of those who stammer this can be a helpful thing to do, but it is not the panacea for everyone.

Consider which of these problems with breathing may contribute to your speaking difficulties:

- *Using your breathing mechanism incorrectly* Do you use your full lung capacity to breathe or only the upper part of your chest? Do you use your diaphragm correctly when breathing? (You may need to get a professional opinion about these aspects of breathing.)
- *Frequency* Do you breathe in too often or too little? Do you try to speak even though you are running out of air?
- *Rushing* Do you take enough time to breathe? Do you gasp for air?
- *Tension* Do you feel tight or tense when you breathe in or when you breathe out? Do you ever feel that you cannot get enough air into your lungs?

Associated tension and movements

As mentioned earlier, one of the strategies some people use to reduce their stammering is to make extra little movements. Unfortunately, while these 'added extras' may work for a time, ultimately they fail to alleviate the difficulties and become enmeshed in the stammer itself. One of us had a client who had so many of these additional behaviours they were more of a problem than the stammer which had precipitated them. He was unable to keep his body still, bounced up and down on his seat, tapped with his feet and hands and frequently hit himself on the thigh and the face. Of course this is an extreme example and for many people the additional movements may be confined to an eye blink, a frowning, wrinkled forehead or a little tap of the toes. Nevertheless, however small the movement, it can still distract the listener and draw attention to the stammer which is trying to be disguised.

Consider which of the following might apply to you when you speak:

- clenching your hands or toes;
- shifting the position of your body a great deal;
- moving your arms and/or legs a lot, say tapping, gesticulating;
- fidgeting or fiddling with an object;
- covering your face or mouth with your hand, hair or clothing;
- jerking your head.

Finally, we would like you to consider which parts of your body are unnecessarily tense when you speak. Many people have the misconception that performing to the best of their ability involves effort and exertion. In actual fact, the reverse is true – you should aim to keep yourself relaxed and the movement or activity should be performed with as little effort as possible. The same principle applies to speaking. Struggling with and pushing out the sounds and words contributes to an increase in the severity of the stammering. For example, tension in the voice box can lead to blocks, while tightness in the chest and/or diaphragm leads to breathing difficulties, and tension in the muscles of speech may produce several problems in articulating sounds.

Consider where the areas of tension are when you speak:

- all over your body – do you hold yourself in a stiff posture when talking to someone?
- in your head, like feelings of increased pressure;
- in your face;
- in your neck and across your shoulders;
- in your stomach and chest;
- in your arms and legs;
- anywhere else?

It may be worth asking a close friend whether or not they notice any tension while you are speaking to them. They can perhaps pick up on things which are not so obvious to you. Because you have become so accustomed to the muscle tightness, you do not notice it.

General communication

Some adults we know have very poor communication even though they are fluent speakers. We also know some adults who stammer who are very good communicators. Indeed, one of our group members won a cup in a public speaking competition. This demonstrates that there is more to good communication skills than fluency alone. Sometimes adults who stammer do not always acknowledge this. They assume that because they stammer, the rest of their communication is disordered too and their listeners see the stammer and only the stammer. In fact, there are a number of skills which make up good communication, which we will discuss in much more detail later. For now we suggest you take a cursory glance at a few, in particular.

Volume We have met people who stammer who had chosen to speak very quietly. When this was discussed with them we realized that they were adopting this way of speaking in an attempt to prevent other people from hearing their stammer. Of course, in reality, their listeners could not hear much of what they were saying and would frequently ask them to repeat or might ignore their contributions altogether.

What do you notice about the volume of your speech? Is it too loud or too quiet? Does it vary to take into account the situation and the level of background noise with which your listener(s) are having to contend?

Pitch With regard to this aspect of communication, we recall one of our clients who used a flat, monotonous voice routinely. He believed this gave him more control over his fluency, but it did nothing to promote his often erudite opinions and frequently sent his listeners to sleep!

In addition to variety of tone, consider whether your pitch is generally too high or too low. The former female prime minister of England attempted to increase her public standing and add weight to her arguments by lowering the pitch of her speaking voice quite dramatically during her years of office. Perhaps there are lessons in this for us all!

Speed There is much written about the speed of speech used by adults who stammer. Some authorities believe there is a link between the lack of ability to make rapid, coordinated muscle movements and stammering. In our experience, we have found that some people can speak faster than others, just as some run quicker than we do! However, it seems more important to identify when your speed causes you to trip or fall over or, in speech terms, to know the speed that is comfortable for you and affords you most fluency.

There is a tendency for some adults who stammer to speed up when they are most fluent. It is almost as if there is an inbuilt fear that, if they do not keep going the 'bogey man of stammers' will catch them and their speech will fall apart. In fact, the reverse may be true. If they keep control of their speed, they are more likely to keep control of their fluency.

We have also noted that some people increase the speed of their speech immediately following a stammer. Using the racing analogy again, it is as if they wish to run away from the moment of stammering, putting as much distance, or speech, between themselves and the stammer as they can.

Consider these issues in relation to your own speech:

- Is the speed with which you speak generally too fast or too slow?
- Do you speed up the more fluent your speech is?
- Do you slow down as you anticipate a stammer?
- Do you speed up immediately after stammering?
- Do you pause enough or are the pauses too long?

Non-verbal aspects Non-verbal behaviours – such as eye contact, facial expression and body posture – are very important features of our total communication and contribute greatly to the messages our listeners pick up. We can betray many of our innermost thoughts and feelings about the person we are talking to, the subject matter of our speech and our reactions to stammering in the non-verbal aspects of communication.

Thinking about stammering in particular, a listener often takes his cue for how to react to a stammer from the way the speaker behaves. If, while blocking or repeating sounds, the speaker looks the listener straight in the eye and carries on speaking, the stammer may well be disregarded and attention focused on the content of what was said. If, however, the block is accompanied by loss of eye contact, looking away and perhaps a shift of body position, the listener's attention is drawn to the stammer and they may realize that the person is embarrassed or uncomfortable and thus react to the stammer in a similarly disconcerted way.

Consider these issues in relation to some of your non-verbal behaviour:

- Do you look away from people when you stammer?
- Do you stare at people when you stammer?
- Do you find it easy or hard to look at people when they are talking to you?
- Does your facial expression match what you are saying?
- Do you show too little or too much expression in your face when talking or listening?
- What do people see in your face when you anticipate stammering, while you are stammering and after the stammer is over?

The internal aspects

There are some people for whom the internal aspects of stammering are more of a problem than its outward display. These people, while regarding themselves as having a stammer, may have a hard time convincing those around them that their speech is a problem. Their partners, friends, colleagues, children and so on do not hear it, so for them it does not happen. However, those with the stammer know that they are doing all sorts of things to prevent the stammer from being observed and heard. In fact, their day-to-day lives may be a constant battleground, a fight to keep the stammer under wraps.

This disguise – including the compromises they make because of their stammer and the feelings stammering arouses – are all part of the internal aspects of stammering.

A famous speech therapist in America called Joseph Sheehan, a man who stammered himself, came up with a wonderful analogy about the relationship

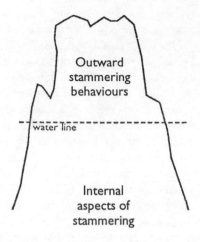

Figure 1 The stammering Iceberg

between the outward stammer and the internal aspects. He said stammering was like an iceberg – the section above the waterline related to the outward stammer (the things other people see and hear), and the part of the iceberg below the water was the internal aspects of stammering (see Figure 1). Thus, any work on modifying stammering should address both parts of the iceberg. It is not enough to change the obvious aspects. Unless the person tackles the less obvious aspects, bringing them to the surface to 'melt', the stammer will never truly be controlled.

When considering what is below the waterline in your stammer, the following should be included.

Avoidances

Once again, Sheehan had something pertinent to say. He categorized avoidance under five main headings:

- Word avoidance.
- Situation avoidance.
- Feeling avoidance.
- Relationship avoidance.

- Behaving as a different kind of person (a sort of avoidance of your true self).

Consider your own avoidances under Sheehan's categories.

Word avoidance Do you:

- change a word to a different one that you think is easier to say?
- alter the order of words?
- pretend you have forgotten a word?
- pretend you have not heard a question?
- create a distraction of some kind, such as coughing or dropping something?
- put on an accent or funny voice to get over a difficult word?
- start off a sentence with a phrase or particular word that you know you can say as a run-in to a feared word?
- add in extra words as a lead-in to saying a specific word on which you think you will stammer?
- choose to remain silent rather than risk saying the word?

Situation avoidance Do you avoid doing particular tasks or activities because you think you will stammer? Examples of frequently avoided situations (reported by our clients) include asking for items in shops, asking directions, using the phone, asking for things which involve queuing, asking for things from someone seated behind a glass partition, going on buses, speaking to people in authority and speaking in groups.

Make a list of the situations or activities you put off or avoid.

Feeling avoidance Because stammering can occur more when expressing certain emotions, a person sometimes avoids this sort of speaking. This can result in others having a false perception of that person. A client of ours, for example, did not thank relatives for presents as he found this disrupted his fluency. He chose therefore to let his family think he did not like the gifts or was rude and ungrateful rather than stammer in front of them. For another client, apologizing was difficult because it made him feel weak, in addition to the undermining effect his stammer had on him. We have also met people who find it hard to express the gentler side of their nature for a similar reason.

You might find it useful to reflect on how you express a range of emotions.

Are there any which you find hard to express? Does your stammer play a part in this?

Relationship avoidance Making and keeping friends places a lot of speaking demands on a person. Initially, you may have to introduce yourself, ask the other person questions about themselves or a topic, answer their questions of you. As the relationship progresses, you have to make an effort to keep the conversation and, ultimately, the relationship going. Perhaps you will have to use the phone to contact them, book tickets, arrange outings, speak to difficult people in their hearing and so on. Your stammer may be apparent sooner or later, and you will have to deal with your own reactions to it in addition to those of the other person. No wonder some people who stammer find themselves avoiding making new friends and stick with relationships which are really dead and buried, or do not do all they might to keep old ones going.

Ask yourself if you ever avoid making or continuing relationships specifically because of your stammer.

Avoidance of your self This one is trickier to explain. If you have big feet or ears that stick out, you would not construe yourself as socially inept. You may not like your feet or your ears particularly and wish they were different, but it would not mean that you viewed yourself as fundamentally inadequate and separate from other people. Somehow, having a stammer can be different from this.

Some people, instead of accepting the stammer as something they do, choose to run away from it or try to hide it. They do not see it as an isolated behaviour, but, rather, it affects their whole view of themselves. They become a 'stammerer' rather than a 'person who speaks in a certain way'.

Do you find yourself doing all you can not to show your stammer? Do you feel ashamed of it and want to sweep it under the carpet? Are you intent on not letting others know about it? What would be the consequence if you no longer fought it but just let it happen? Would people actually see you more negatively as you fear? Would you stammer less or more? Would you do more or less of the things you would like to? We will address this aspect in more detail later.

Feelings

There are a number of other internal aspects of stammering which are worthy of a mention. We would like to discuss in particular several emotions which our clients have frequently discussed with us (some additional ones will be addressed later in the book).

Anxiety First, we would like you to consider the level of anxiety you experience when talking. Now we are not discussing here the day-to-day stress and strain of everyday living. Certainly, in these days of increasing pressure from a variety of sources, all of us will experience some degree of tension and anxiety from time to time. In relation to stammering, though, we are particularly concerned with anxiety that is felt in speaking situations – the telephone, a presentation at work, reading bedtime stories to the children or whatever.

You might find it useful in your continuing attempts to identify and confront the different aspects of your stammer to consider the level of anxiety you feel in speaking situations. Are there some situations which evoke more anxiety than others? How is the anxiety realized? What do you do to control it? Are the controlling mechanisms effective in every case? When do they work and what can you learn from the occasions when they do work which will help you in the future?

Isolation One thing which many clients have reported to us are the feelings of loneliness and isolation which having a stammer brings. This might be because stammering is fundamentally a breakdown in communication, perhaps because it is not yet an issue which is readily discussed or because of society's attitude to it. Whatever the reason, it does not have to be an event which separates and alienates you from others.

Many of our clients have gained much from becoming members of a local self-help group and/or the British Stammering Association, but we will discuss this in greater detail in Chapter 8. We recall one client who had never met another person who stammered before. As luck would have it, the Leeds self-help group was hosting an open day after our initial session with him and it was suggested that he might like to attend. We saw him early in the day at the back of the hall looking rather lost. Later that same day he was to be found in animated conversation with several members of the local group and we understand the discussion adjourned to a nearby hostelry for several additional hours! In a subsequent therapy session, he commented that the day had changed his life. Having not met a single person who stammered and then to be faced with a whole hall full of them, sharing his problems and difficulties, was 'mind blowing', he said.

Compromises

In life we all have to make compromises. Some we may not mind too much, others allow us to live in harmony with people we care about, while some can be difficult to live with and deny something basic in us. In our clinics we have both had conversations with people whose lives have been shaped by the

25

compromises they have made because of their stammer. One client chose not to ask the girl he loved to marry him, another feared job interviews because his speech was so dysfluent and decided to study instead. Allowing your stammer to shape your life can be a soul-destroying path to take. There is always the knowledge that you could have done X if only . . . . Getting control of your stammer can often mean taking control of your life and saying 'I am going to do X even if I do stammer'. Life will be more fulfilling as a result.

As part of therapy, we often ask people to write a description of their stammer so detailed that it allows us to learn to stammer in their particular way. What follows are a couple of such descriptions which we hope will illustrate both the benefits of this exercise and the individuality of people's stammers.

Stammering like Bryan

When I stammer it can be in a variety of different ways. It can be phrases or just parts of words, and they are either effortless or quite tense hard blocks. They are usually quite short (one or two seconds) and are mainly in the mouth or throat. On longer blocks I sometimes move my arms and legs when I get into the block, and I can get very tense in my body. To relieve these hard blocks I try and relax the tension in my body and sometimes I insert sounds, like m and n before the word I am blocking on.

When I am in a hard block, I can feel very tense in certain parts of my body – these are mainly my arms and legs, my chest, stomach and face. During a bad block, my jaw and mouth can lock in an open position, while I try and say the word. Also, I sometimes momentarily look away from the person I am talking to.

When I am in a difficult speaking situation, I tend to speak too quickly and get faster as I talk. This results in taking too few pauses and running out of breath while I am talking. After I have been talking for a while, I can feel short of breath and tired.

For some of the time when I stammer it will be effortless and the fact that I stammered does not really bother me. However, when I have bad blocks I feel frustrated and angry at myself for not being able to say the words fluently. I sometimes feel inadequate and inferior to fluent people, and dissatisfied with the way I talk and the way I feel I come across to other people. When I am more concerned with the way I am speaking, rather than what I am saying, this can have the effect of making me feel uncomfortable, therefore increasing any tension I may have. This then makes me more cautious about speaking in situations when I know that I will probably stammer.

Bryan Wood

Stammering like Diane

This manual will provide you with precise knowledge on how to be a proficient stammerer. By completing this manual you will be able to recognize that stammering is a complex condition that takes endurance and great skill to master. The beginning stammerer must be willing to use endless amounts of mental energy and to accept personality change in order to become a professional stammerer.

As a beginner you must first learn to be always conscious that you are a stammerer to enable yourself to be prepared for any situation that may arise. It may be frustrating at first because you may only stammer mildly in the beginning, but do not be discouraged. In no time at all you will develop a severe problem. To assist you in achieving this objective I have devised a number of rules which must be followed.

RULE 1

Accept the fact that if you stammer it will create a significant personality change. This is an essential part of being a proficient stammerer. Every good stammerer must adapt to a personality change. You must learn to become passive in many situations, which may include pretending to be an indecisive, uninformed person. Also, to accompany this, you will need to have feelings of being overwhelmed, depressed, anxious, fatigued and inadequate. These feelings will not develop at first but with practice and dedication to your stammer you will achieve your goals.

RULE 2

Remember always to avoid any situation you may have difficulty with in order to build your fear to a maximum level. Start out by avoiding situations such as speaking in front of large crowds and gradually build yourself up to avoiding most situations where you have to talk. (Do not include social situations when you are able to talk as you please.) This will eventually rule your life and you will definitely be on your way to being a professional stammerer.

Here are some guidelines on avoidance:

- If you can put things in writing rather than speaking take advantage of that opportunity. It is the only time you will get to express yourself without tension.

27

- Never use the telephone unless it is absolutely necessary. If you need to make an appointment, drive to where you need to go and waste all of your time.
- Never make new friends unless they live alone. In this way you can be sure that your new friend will be the only person answering the telephone when you ring.
- Alternatively, establish a relationship of some kind with everyone in the home you are phoning so they know your voice when you ring. This will prevent you from having to ask for the person you wish to speak to by name.
- Never order what you want when going to a restaurant to eat. Only order what you can say. If you cannot say anything, just get the same dish as the person sitting next to you. (Hopefully your tastes will be the same.) A useful tip: having some wine before you actually have to sit down and order may put you at ease and you may even be able to order for yourself.
- While working, never take the initiative to answer phones and avoid taking any new information that needs to be passed on. In order to keep your job, you must be a hard worker to compensate for your speech. Keep very busy and most people will not notice you.
- Last, but not least, try to avoid most career advancements that will require you to be articulate, even if there is a pay increase. Know your limitations!

RULE 3

When you are unable to avoid situations, communicate in whatever way possible, even if you appear incompetent.

Word substitutions and backtracking are your best friends. They will enable you to speak fluently when all else fails. Be aware that when you appear incompetent to others this will cause feelings of embarrassment, low self-esteem and depression, but at least you can speak! Try to repress these feelings to avoid them ruining your life.

You will be able to use word substitution in most social situations and in some formal ones. The only problem will arise when you cannot substitute words. In those cases you will have to remove yourself as soon as possible in order to cope with the situation.

RULE 4

You may experience short periods of fluency. When this occurs, take advantage and get things accomplished.

Make all appointments and enquiries on this day but be sure not to follow up on most of them. This ensures that people think you are irresponsible and disinterested.

These are the four major rules that must be followed to perfect a stammer. You must be a quick thinker and a strong-willed character to carry out this torture upon yourself. I have added some extra 'hints' to assist you.

- If you are fluent for one sentence, get everything out you want to say in that one sentence. However, beware as most of the time you will have to repeat what you said because the rate makes it impossible to understand. Do not be downhearted. Take the chance whenever the opportunity arises.
- Pretend not to hear someone when they ask you your name. If the worst comes to the worst, say whatever name you can say. Who will know (aside from you, of course)?
- Make excuses for not ringing people.
- Make the least eye contact possible when a block is evident. It eases the pressure.
- Backtrack while talking. Most people get so confused, the attention is taken away from yourself.
- Procrastinate when phone calls are a must.
- Place phrases in front of a sentence to get you started.
- Cough or yawn as a distraction.
- Never slow down. You will block ten times more than you normally would.
- Wear a name tag for formal interviews to lessen the pressure. (Forget to take it off for a day or two.)
- If you cannot *say* your name, spell it out to people.
- Never sit by the phone.
- Never forget how easy your life would be if you did not have a stammer.

Diane Buckle

Summary

In this chapter we have asked you, the person who stammers, to look as objectively as possible at your stammer. We have suggested examining small pieces of it at a time, as it can be hard to see the whole picture in one go and also because it can be difficult to confront something which is painful and

29

that, consequently, you avoid. We are aware that each stammer is individual and we would like to emphasize that only parts of this chapter may be relevant to you. Nevertheless, we recommend that you consider all the sections and then choose which to concentrate your efforts on.

For more fluent speakers, we hope that this chapter will have given you an insight into the complexity of stammering and a realization that all you see – and hear, in this case – is not the whole picture.

3
Why me?

From reading Chapter 1 or, perhaps, from seeing statistics about stammering elsewhere, you will be aware that approximately 5 children in every 100 stammer, while only 1 of these 5 still stammers in adulthood. If you are close to someone who stammers, you will probably wonder why that is. If you stammer yourself, we guess you would like to know why you ended up as that one and not one of the other four. You will probably often have asked yourself, 'Why me?' Indeed, this same question is likely to have been asked by many people with any 'problem' they wish they did not have. The question may be about something different ('Why am I fat/spotty/short/ freckly/disabled/short-sighted/hopeless at languages?' and so on), but the feeling behind it is similar. It is also a question speech and language therapists ask about their clients – why is it *this* child and not *that* one who will stammer when they grow up? From Chapter 1 you will also realize that the short answer is 'We don't know yet'. The long answer is what this chapter is all about!

Before we start to try and answer the question in the best way that current understanding allows, let's look for a moment at why you might want to know the answer. We can hazard a few guesses. It may be because:

- you and/or your parents were told as a child that you would 'grow out of it', but you didn't and you want to know why;
- you feel that by gaining some insight, your speech will improve;
- you have children and want to ensure they do not have to suffer as you have;
- you wish you could find something or someone to blame for your stammer;
- you have heard conflicting theories in the past and these have not helped your understanding of stammering;
- like us, you are curious;
- you have begun stammering as an adult and want to know why.

Whatever the reason, we hope we can provide you with at least some understanding. What we say may not fulfil all your expectations (we don't think, for example, that knowing more about it will make you fluent). Neither do we claim to have *the* answer but merely a way of helping us to make sense of this incredibly complicated problem. We hope it helps you, too. We do not propose to go into a great deal of detail as this book is primarily aimed to help you at the stage you are at now. If you want to find out more about how stammering can develop in children, reading our book *Helping Children Cope with Stammering* (Sheldon Press, 1996) covers this area in detail.

Speech and language therapists also want to understand 'why?' Here are some of our own reasons for this:

- We want an explanation which makes sense to us, especially as so little is known about the original cause.
- We would really like to predict with certainty which four children out of the five will *not* go on to stammer so we can concentrate our time and efforts on the one who will.
- Understanding how a child moves from having dysfluent speech to having a full-blown stammer can give us more ideas about how we may help prevent the same happening to another child. This in turn will help us deal more effectively with that particular child, hopefully preventing some of the anguish stammering can create. The whole purpose of our work is to be therapeutic, so the answer to the question may ultimately help us reduce the incidence of stammering to 1 in 200, 2,000 or reduce it even further.
- Finally, let's face it, we are also immensely curious – we want so much to understand anything and everything about the nature of the problem that can create so much unhappiness and leads to clients coming to us for help.

Developmental and acquired stammering

By far the most common scenario is that stammering is developmental. That is, it starts in childhood and changes and develops as the child grows. It frequently ceases altogether, as we have seen from the statistics, or it can stay fairly constant or become increasingly severe, in each case with or without therapy.

A study of children growing up in Newcastle upon Tyne, the results of which were published in the 1960s, showed that stammering most frequently developed between the ages of two and five and that onset after the age of nine was relatively uncommon. More unusually still, stammering can start later in life. In these cases there is often an associated illness affecting the brain, such as Parkinson's disease or some damage to the brain, as can occur after a stroke or with a head injury. Sometimes it can follow a psychological trauma and, indeed, there were several reported cases of stammering following 'shell shock' in the two world wars. In addition, there are a number of people who appear to have acquired a stammer in adulthood for an unknown reason. However, these occurrences are rare.

As stammering most usually develops in childhood, we shall now spend some time looking at how this may happen.

The developmental stages of stammering

We will look briefly at three stages of stammering which many people are likely to have been through since the onset of their stammering. These we call:

- Early dysfluency.
- Borderline stammering.
- Confirmed stammering.

Early dysfluency

If you listen to the speech of any young child, you will soon become aware that it is often far from fluent. Most children hesitate, repeat, revise and stumble over words as they seek to find the best way to express their ideas and feelings. This dysfluency tends to be more apparent when they are tired, ill, upset or excited. It is very hard to differentiate this 'normal' non-fluency from the early stages of stammering.

Most developmental stammering starts between the ages of two and a half and five. At this early stage, children are usually completely unaware and unconcerned about their speech. Adults around them may, however, be worried, especially if they know someone else who stammers or, indeed, if they stammer themselves. It is common for adults to look ahead, to see the stammer not as it is for children but as it might be if they were adults.

Although there is no 'blueprint', as it were, that we can use to differentiate normal dysfluency from early stammering, there are some areas speech and language therapists find it helpful to look at as they try to work out if a child is at risk of stammering. To illustrate this more clearly, we will take the examples of two imaginary dysfluent children. We will endeavour to see if we can discover any factors which can help us predict whether or not they will go on to stammer or will become fluent.

Sam

Sam is a boy of two and a half. He lives with his Mum, Dad and brother, Billy, who is nearly six. His Mum works from 9.30 am to 5 pm, three days a week. His Dad works full time and does three different weekly shifts. Mum takes Billy to her workplace nursery on the days she is working and he stays at home with her the rest of the time. He's been at the nursery since he was one and really enjoys it.

Sam can be rather a clumsy child – he falls over a lot and his co-ordination is a little immature. He doesn't sleep too well at the best of times – he never seems to goes to sleep before 9 o'clock at night and then, of course, he's bleary eyed in the morning! It's a bit of a rush on the days that Mum is working and if Dad has been working nights, too, it can be rather fraught in the morning, trying to get ready for school. Sometimes if Sam's speech is very dysfluent when his Mum is trying to get ready, it is very frustrating for her to wait for him to finish what he is saying and on occasions she tells him to hurry up and 'spit it out' or carries on rushing round as he is talking and admits to not really listening.

Sam's Dad used to stammer when he was younger and still does sometimes, although he manages to hide it most of the time. He tells Sam to repeat words he stumbles over and Sam usually says them fluently the second time. Both Sam's parents try to make sure he gets some individual attention from each of them as often as possible. Sam has been speaking for quite a while and his language skills are very good – he uses quite complicated sentences. He isn't aware of having any difficulty in talking and his parents describe him as a 'real chatterbox'.

Some factors which we think might make stammering more likely for Sam

These are that he is:

- a boy – more boys than girls stammer;
- not getting enough rest;
- feeling rushed;
- not being listened to or looked at when he is talking;
- being told to 'spit it out' – raising Sam's awareness can make him concerned about speech and increase his dysfluency;
- a relative of someone with a stammer;
- clumsy and so may have poor muscle control.

Some factors which we think might make stammering less likely for Sam

He:

- has a stable home background;
- has started to speak early and has good language skills – although this can sometimes act as a disadvantage if the child is too concerned about saying things 'just right';
- enjoys talking;
- is getting quality time with his parents;

- lacks awareness of any speaking difficulty.

Lucy

Lucy is just four years old. She is the longed-for girl, the youngest of five children. The eldest is a boy of 14. There is a lot of noise in the household and someone is always holding forth about something! Lucy's speech skills are a bit delayed for her age, but then she really doesn't need to talk much as there is always someone to anticipate her needs. She only has to point and someone will get her a drink, a biscuit or whatever it is she wants. It's quite hard to get a 'turn' to talk anyway, someone always butts in! Her parents and grand-parents adore her and find her 'stammer' rather appealing; in fact, they sometimes mimic her in fun as they think it is so cute. No one ever corrects her speech. Everyone likes to talk to her. She gets asked a lot of questions, although often she has hardly begun to think of an answer to one before the next one is asked. Her grandparents collect her from the playgroup she goes to three times a week and as soon as they see her, it's one question after another – 'Did you have a nice time?', 'Who did you play with?', 'Was Susie there?', 'Did you drink up your milk?', you know the kind of thing. She gets asked to 'perform' a lot, too – 'Sing Humpty Dumpty' and so on – and sometimes she really doesn't want to.

Lucy's Dad is worried about redundancies his firm could be announcing soon, as money is tight at the best of times. Maybe this is one of the reasons her Mum and Dad haven't been getting on so well lately – there's been a lot of shouting. They've tried to shield the children from their difficulties, but, inevitably, the children must have noticed at times and everyone's been a bit edgy.

Lucy spends most Fridays with her other Grandad. They have a lovely time together and he gives her a lot of 'space', letting her choose what to do. He listens to her and always gives her time to say the things she wants. It's a very special time for them both.

Lucy sleeps well – her Mum says 'she doesn't take any rocking'.

Some factors which we think might make stammering more likely for Lucy

These include:

- her delayed speech and language development;
- a noisy household where it is hard to get a turn to speak;
- being interrupted;

- being mimicked;
- being asked a lot of questions;
- being asked to 'perform';
- tension in the household.

Some factors which we think might make stammering less likely for Lucy
These are that:

- she is a girl – more boys than girls stammer and girls who do stammer tend to recover from it more frequently than boys;
- her speech is not corrected;
- she gets plenty of sleep;
- she is getting 'quality time' with her Grandad;
- she lacks awareness of any speaking difficulty.

Can we say who will stammer at this stage?
Unfortunately these points are only part of the story. Those we have listed are just some of the relevant factors. In addition, although we can say that there are some areas of concern for both Sam and Lucy, we cannot make a valid prediction about whether or not they will stammer because we do not yet know the answers to the following questions:

- Why does the speech of some children but not others become disrupted even when there are apparently similar factors which apply?
- Are the factors which make stammering more likely or those which make it less likely the most relevant ones? Or do they cancel each other out?
- Are there other factors we have not considered or discovered? For example, could there be a stammering gene? Is environment more or less important than heredity? Is the child's temperament important?
- Where is the balance? How many factors do there need to be to tip a child towards either stammering or fluency?

Borderline stammering

This is the next developmental stage. For a child to move to this stage, certain of the following changes will happen but they may not all occur in one child.

How the child views their speech
The most important of these changes is the way the child feels or thinks about their dysfluent speech. If you remember, the child in the early dysfluency stage was either unaware of any difficulty with talking or unconcerned about their speech, although it might frustrate them for a moment if they took too

long to say what they wanted. The borderline stammering child, though, begins to have some awareness or concern about this.

It could be because they start to be aware that their speech is not exactly as they would like or that it doesn't feel like it is under their control. It may be because the reactions of other people indicate that something is not quite right – they tell them to slow down, take it easy, take a deep breath and so on or they give more subtle clues like looking away for a moment or tensing up when the dysfluency occurs.

The way the child behaves

Because the child starts to view their speech negatively, they may start to behave differently. Sometimes a child acts more introverted, talks less, becomes more awkward to deal with, changes the things they do after school (for example, they stop calling on their friends and instead play alone on the computer), answers fewer questions in class, doesn't volunteer for things that involve talking and so on – the possibilities are endless. We expect some of you may be able to recall some of these or other changes you made at this stage in your stammer, as you became aware that your speech was 'not quite right' or acceptable to others.

The way speech sounds

Changes can occur in any or all of the following areas:

- *The amount of dysfluency.* The child's speech can become more noticeably dysfluent at this stage – the stammer can occur more often or the moments of stammering may last longer.
- *The type of dysfluency* Another change which can occur at this stage is that there is more tension in the child's stammering. Perhaps, for example, they start to block, rather than repeat sounds in a relaxed way.
- *Where and when the child is dysfluent* Because this stage is characterized by increased awareness, sometimes the child starts to anticipate stammering with specific people and in situations they perceive to be difficult. The dysfluency can therefore start to be more apparent in such situations, for example, with strangers, teachers, in the school term rather than the holidays and so on.
- *The use of devices to hide the dysfluency* As the child's awareness of difficulty in speaking grows, so they may start to try to hide their dysfluency. They do this in a number of ways. They perhaps change an occasional word, pretend they have forgotten an answer, put in an extra word or phrase to disguise the difficulty they are experiencing or make the

feared word easier to run into. We shall not list all the ways of hiding stammering as this list, as we are sure you know from experience, is fairly long!

- *Extra movements of the face or body* In an attempt to force the difficult word out, the child uses more tension than usual. This can result in visible movements of the face or body, such as screwing up the eyes, pushing together the tongue, lips and roof of the mouth, pushing with the leg and so on. These movements may then become incorporated into the stammer.

Other people's reactions

Sometimes people give the child advice – slow down, take a deep breath, say it again, think before you speak and so on. This can have the effect of making the child more aware of a problem which was perhaps not a problem to them originally. Other people react with a 'conspiracy of silence' – they avoid mentioning of the dysfluency at all costs so it is just not talked about. If the child has become aware and concerned about the stammer, they may begin to feel that these people are not mentioning it because they do not want to upset them. If this is the case, they may feel that they should keep the problem to themselves and then they have no one to share it with. This is when feelings of isolation can start. The child may even begin to believe that it is not talked about because it is shameful and unacceptable and so they feel the need to hide it even more.

Parents and others have a difficult role. If they bring the stammer to the child's notice by suggesting ways of controlling it or by talking about it as a problem when it is not one for the child, they risk creating a problem where none existed previously. If, however, they avoid mentioning it and the child is aware, they can encourage the child to view it negatively. It is not an easy course to steer. You may wish to reflect on what happened in your own case and on why others might have reacted in the ways they did.

Confirmed stammering

The biggest change that will have taken place for someone to have reached this stage is that they now see themselves as a stammerer, rather than as a person who, among many other things, happens to have a stammer. The stammer is at the front of their mind for much of the time. It plays a large part in decisions made regarding such things as career and social activities. It is likely that this is the stage you have now reached. Although we have called it 'confirmed' stammering, it does not mean there is nothing which can be done to change it. If that were the case there would be little point in our writing any more in this book. Something that is confirmed can always be cancelled – a party, train ticket, wedding, but the work involved is likely to be greater than it would be if the booking – or the stammer – is at a less advanced stage. As you will see, the rest of the book is devoted to looking at practical ways in which you can help yourself or get help from others.

Before we do that, though, let's look at a few of the factors involved in confirmed stammering. As you read, see how each of these applies to you.

The stammer itself

This may or may not become more severe. Sometimes the struggle involved in trying to get words out intensifies, resulting in the stammer becoming more noticeable to others. Not only can the struggle affect the intensity of the actual speech, but the accompanying movements of head and/or body may also become greater. One person may jerk back their head in an attempt to force the words out when they get stuck, another may tap their foot or clench their fists. Breathing often becomes disrupted, with the person running out of breath or controlling their air supply in an ineffective way, making their speech sound jerky or resulting in its being of a low volume.

The stammer may, however, 'go underground'. In these cases the person becomes so adept at hiding and avoiding it that they hardly ever stammer openly. The stammer is a well-guarded secret that they keep from everyone, even sometimes those closest to them.

Negative feelings about stammering

Many and various negative emotions can become associated with the stammer. These include embarrassment, fear, shame, anger, sadness – the list goes on. These feelings can be very potent and affect all areas of the person's life. Very often, because of the reactions of others or because of the constraints the person puts on themselves, they learn to view stammering as something they *are*, not just something they *do*. It can become so much a part of them that, as one of our clients once said, 'I do not know any more where my stammer ends and I begin'. We will explore these feelings in greater detail in later chapters.

Attempts to hide the stammer

An important development at this stage is that the person feels so negatively about their stammer that they attempt to hide it wherever and whenever possible. Confirmed stammering always involves avoidance to a lesser or greater degree. Joseph Sheehan, an American speech and language therapist, lists five different levels of avoidance that we discussed in Chapter 1, which are word, situation, feeling, relationship and self role.

Behaving like a different kind of person

One of the things we are often told by people who stammer is that they feel trapped. Because they often try whenever possible to disguise or hide the stammer, they come across differently from the way they feel they really are. They may, for example, choose to let other people think they are shy when they say little, unintelligent or forgetful because they do not give the answers to questions, unassertive because they do not give their opinions and so on. Stammering can be viewed so negatively that people would prefer others to think of them in these ways than let them know that they stammer. Is this the case for you?

Letting the stammer take the blame for failures

If we have a problem it is all too common for us to blame it for many of our difficulties. The two of us are both struggling to learn to play musical instruments. We blame lack of time to practise for our poor progress. In fact, we choose to organize our time in a particular way (writing books instead of practising, for example!). We may also need to face up to the fact that we are not inherently musical, have taken up playing relatively late in life, are not prepared to study the theory as well as the practical aspects, and so on. So it is with stammering. Perhaps you need to look at other reasons for things not going as you would have liked – you did not get a particular job because you were not the best candidate, your girlfriend or boyfriend ended your relationship because they did not think you were compatible, you did not give a good talk because you did not prepare sufficiently – rather than these things happening solely because you stammer. It is not easy for any of us to face up to some of the truths about ourselves we would rather ignore, but if we want to move forward, we need to do just that. We are not underestimating the courage it takes to confront your stammer, just pointing out that such a difficult and honest approach may be needed if you are to make progress.

Summary

In this chapter we have looked at how stammering can develop from a disruption of speech which is of little or no concern to a young child, to a debilitating disorder which affects all aspects of a person's life. We have also noted that, although there are other ways, this is the most common way stammering can start.

If you stammer yourself, we hope you have been able to relate this to your own experience and now have a little more understanding of how you may have reached your current situation.

WHY ME?

If you are reading this book because you know someone who stammers or are just interested in the subject, we hope you will have had some of your queries answered, too.

4

So you want to change?

If you have a stammer, we must presume that you are reading this book in the hope that it will help to change the way you speak or, perhaps, the way you feel about yourself as a communicator.

In this chapter we consider change in fairly general terms before we go on to look at changes in speech in particular. Our life experiences would seem to tell us that some things are easier to change than others, perhaps depending on the degree of importance we place on them. The more important things are usually harder to change. For example, it may be easy to eat different types of sandwiches every day at work because you enjoy eating different foods and because you believe it is important to vary your diet. It might be harder to change your lunchtime eating habits and eat the same type of sandwich daily as it would be boring and would not fit in with your view of what healthy eating is. In other words, there are some activities and feelings which are more difficult to change because somehow they incorporate part of what you believe about yourself.

In one group therapy session, we were all experimenting with change and the group decided that one of us should experiment with changing our appearance. It was decreed that earrings should not be worn for a week. The challenge was accepted, albeit reluctantly, although at that stage it was not clear what the source of the unwillingness to do this was. During the week that followed it was noticed that more distinctive combinations of colours and clothes were chosen. It was as if the lack of earrings was being compensated for in some way. Having thought about this, it became clear that the earrings had become a sort of statement of individuality and when this form of expression was removed, then some alternative way of making a statement developed.

These examples illustrate that change can be quite a complicated issue. How much more complicated, then, it is likely to be when what you want to change is something that you have been doing for a lifetime and feel you have little or no control over.

How do you get to the point of wanting to make a change?

There are perhaps a number of issues to consider here. Let us look at them in turn.

External factors

Society

First, there is the society in which we live. Society often tells a person who stammers that their speech is unacceptable. As we have noted previously, the stereotypical view of stammering is often of a nervous, anxious person who lacks assertion and drive, although there are some signs that this is changing. It is not helped, however, by media portrayal of humorous halfwits with chips up their noses, sex-starved, mean-minded grocers or psychopathic, violent individuals, all with stammers.

Perhaps for some people the way stammering is portrayed, coupled with a general view that society responds negatively to those who stammer, will encourage the desire for change.

Life events

Second, think about specific events in your life which may stimulate you into action. A common one is marriage. We often have people coming along to our clinics – sometimes for the first time, sometimes not having had therapy for years – who have marriage vows to say and need reassurance and some techniques to get them through the ceremony. There are also those who are anticipating the arrival of children or whose children are beginning to speak. In these instances, there is often a fear that the child will imitate the adult's pattern of speech and begin to stammer as a result.

These life events also put the individual under pressure. The adult with a child wants to have greater control over their own speech, not so much for themselves but because of their child. Perhaps there is a worry that they will let the child down in some way or that the child itself will be disadvantaged because, for example, they never heard a bedtime story being read fluently.

Specific pressures

Next, consider pressures that are exerted from specific sources. These, too, can encourage change.

We have had some cases where a client reports that other people have pressurized them into seeking help. Partners, parents and other family members exert their influence. Occasionally there are those outside the family who are instrumental in getting someone to come along to our clinics. James, for example, came along to a group because his boss had suggested he should seek help. James himself did not at that time feel he had a problem, but responded to his boss's request.

In our experience, it is unusual to meet someone who is seeking help purely because another person suggested it, even though that other person may well be very influential in their life. Usually it is the person concerned who has realized that there is an issue which needs to be addressed. This leads us nicely on to internal pressures.

Internal factors

When we were thinking about this area, we recalled reasons individuals had given us for wanting to come for therapy. People talk, often quite passionately, about the following kinds of motivations.

Having had enough

Life, they say, has become so full of restricted choices, loss of opportunity, unacceptable compromises and sacrifices that they feel they really have to do something.

Importance or saliency

People think about how important the stammer is or has become in their lives. They may say that their speech has become the most important thing in their life. It is frequently on their mind, so that they often evaluate situations in terms of how well they will speak, even when speaking might be a very small part of the whole event. They think about what words or sounds to say and whether they will be able to say them or choose to avoid the word and insert another.

From a therapeutic point of view, we think that, before embarking on major change, the person undertaking it needs to believe some fundamental things about themselves:

- They should believe that they are capable of change. They should not see the process as a lost cause before they have started. The 'Oh, I've tried to change my speech before and it didn't work then' syndrome is quite destructive. They have predicted the outcome even before the starting gun has sounded, so chances are, their own prophecy will then come true.
- They should believe that the outcome is desirable. If, for example, the person feels that slowing their speech down makes them sound too considered, less spontaneous, they will certainly not use a technique like that when situations demand spontaneity. However, it becomes even more of a problem when spontaneity is construed by someone as being an important part of the person they believe themselves to be. Then, talking in this new way becomes a major threat to their self-image. This is why most of the therapy undertaken these days is negotiated between the therapist and the client. This ensures that the steps taken in therapy are small enough to be achievable and not so large as to produce major anxieties and difficulties they cannot cope with.

- Finally, the adult with a stammer should believe that their therapist has what is known in the field of psychology as 'communicator credibility', which means that they feel the therapist knows what they are on about, or at least gives the impression that they do! Using well-respected role models to convey messages in the media is a recognized way of getting the message across effectively. That is why Gary Linekar was portrayed eating a certain brand of crisp and Vinny Jones was not! Thus, those who come to us for therapy in Leeds may be surprised at some of the things they are asked to try out. But if they have a basic belief that we know what we are doing and there are good reasons behind their being asked to do these things, then they are more likely to go along with the suggestions and there is likely to be a more successful outcome than would otherwise be the case. If you choose to go for therapy, of whatever type, then make sure you have a basic belief in and respect for the therapist. If you do not, then any message they may have for you will fall on deaf ears.

Difficulties associated with change

For some reason, most of us do not respond well to the prospect of change in our lives, even though it seems to be the normal pattern of life these days. Why do we find change difficult?

We suggest that there are three main categories of causes of difficulty, which are:

- Practicalities.
- Other people.
- Maintaining the change.

Practicalities

The habit factor

As noted earlier, it is often hard to change simple things but even harder to change things that have been part of our lives for over 20 years or more. Speaking is a process that has developed since childhood and, like other basic functions, such as walking and eating, it is very difficult to break it down and re-establish it in a new pattern.

The 'me' factor

Some people view stammering as part of them. Like the earrings turned out to be in our earlier example, stammering is seen by many as a statement of who they are. As a result, it can be very difficult to change as it may be tied in with other important things individuals believe about themselves. This brings to mind a man we met some years ago when we taught 'slowed speech' technique to many of our clients. This man, who we shall call Brendan, had shown that he could use the technique very effectively in clinic and, unlike many, had managed to make it sound quite normal and acceptable to others who heard him. However, he was choosing *not* to use it in other situations outside therapy sessions. When asked why this was, Brendan replied, 'It does not feel like me'. This led us to think about how, for many people, therapy should be about changing aspects of their thinking, their attitudes to speaking and their views of themselves as communicators in addition to changing the way they speak.

The time factor

As we mentioned before, desperately wanting to change may not be enough. If there are other things going on in your life which are taking up time and mean that you do not have space and/or energy to devote to working on your speech, then we would recommend that you wait until your situation has become easier.

Michael

Michael came to see us two years ago with a moderate stammer that was causing him problems at work and socially. He knew it was restricting him and reducing his choices. We decided to work on some controlling techniques, but we made very little progress. He was made redundant, subsequently started a new job, moved house and became a Dad for the second time. Michael found he did not have any spare capacity to work on his speech and really was doing pretty well in the circumstances just to keep going.

We are not suggesting from this, however, that just because you move house you can't work on changing your speech. People's capacities are different. There are some superhumans around who could have coped with all Michael's changes and worked on new speaking techniques as well. As an individual, you have to consider what *you* are able to take on and cope with.

The saliency factor

By this we mean, is it important enough? Because changing the way you speak can be difficult, you have to be able to make it your top priority, or at least a priority for a while. In Leeds, we ask adults to commit themselves to therapy for about a year. As will be discussed in greater detail later, this is because we believe that changes made over a period of time are likely to be maintained more effectively. However, a year is a long time to keep speech at the top of your agenda and inevitably other issues will intrude. Where possible, we ask that these are set aside to enable the work on speech and related matters to go ahead.

The compromises

If the way a person speaks is an important part of them, then changing that aspect will inevitably involve making compromises of some kind. Some adults we have met have discussed these sacrifices. Adrian talked about how his stammer was related to his individuality. It was something which set him apart from the crowd and that people remembered. Gaining more control over his speech meant that some of that sense of being different was lost. Others have talked about how gaining more control over their stammer has brought about changes in their roles. For example, a person may discover that they can no longer hide behind their problematical speech and will opt out of taking the lead in situations. They may find that they have to be more assertive in the face of perceived wrongdoing and cannot ask others to act and speak for them. These are hard compromises to make and, for some people, it is easier not to make the changes.

Other people

We do not live in a vacuum. We live in a society with its own standards and attitudes towards communication and we interact with people on a daily basis. These other important people in our lives expect us to behave and respond to them in a certain way. They get used to us being a certain type of person and acting in a particular way. If we change and act differently, it can cause, at the very least, some curiosity and, at the most, threat. 'I like you just the way you are. Your stammering does not bother me.' Implicit in such statements is a relationship based on the status quo. Change the status quo and it could mean a change in roles and a different relationship. Vera, with her new speech techniques to practise, did not want her partner to order for her in a restaurant or get her drinks from the bar. Her partner saw this as Vera asserting left-wing tendencies and wanted to know what was going on. For Dick greater speech fluency meant he could choose to go out to work and his wife was no longer the major breadwinner. The question of who then looked after the children became a major source of conflict between them and one which was not easily resolved.

Other people are important, and because they are they need to be informed and involved in the change process. People will require explanations and, usually, once they understand and have a rationale for differences in behaviour or responses, they can cope with them and learn to move with the changes themselves.

Maintaining change

The actual change itself may not be the problem, but keeping it going can be. Whether for management consultants or stammerers, intensive residential courses often produce quite dramatic results. However, after the course, when a person returns to their workplace and faces all the old problems, situations and personalities, they can find that it is hard to keep the newly learnt behaviours going and easier to slip back into old familiar ways.

In Leeds, over a period of 15 years we have tried out different types of therapy programmes with our adult clients. We have run intensive weekend courses with less intensive follow-up sessions. There have been week-long courses with some intensive weekends and regular weekly meetings. The intensive programmes produced quite dramatic changes for most people, but these proved to be relatively short-term ones and clients frequently complained some six months later that change was not maintained and that their control over their speech was decreasing. The less intensive courses have, as you might expect, produced a slower rate of change, but the group members report that they have been able to maintain them well. These experiences are, in fact, mirrored by the research findings in other areas. In weight-loss programmes, in the control of alcohol and substance abuse, researchers have found that change is easier to maintain when it is made slowly over time. It seems that people need to become accustomed to the differences change makes in their lives, learn to live with it and build on it in a gradual way. (Other people involved in their lives also need time to get used to change.) Too much change too quickly is harder to manage and make sense of.

It is very rewarding to look back over the last five years and recall the faces of people who struggled with change and eventually moved on to live more fulfilling lives. Alan, a security officer, began by wanting to sell his house, car and everything in exchange for fluency and ended up accepting his speech and training as a youth worker. Martin arrived for therapy when life was pretty much at its lowest ebb and is now embarking on a psychology degree as a mature student. We are not, like writers of some programmes, claiming this will happen to all who come to our clinics, but certainly for some people it was the right time, it was important enough and they made significant changes.

So how do people change?

So here you are. You want to change very badly, you believe it is the right time, you have enough energy and time to commit yourself to working at it and you have made sure that the important people in your life want to be involved. What are you going to do? How are you going to go about making this change? Where do you start?

Unfortunately, this is not an easy question and it is one which has been the subject of several theories, numerous models and years of research in the field of psychology!

Arising out of a number of theories in the 1960s came the view that attitudes were the key, that the way a person thought and evaluated behaviour actually influenced the way they behaved. Thus, it followed that it was possible to change a person's behaviour by trying to modify their attitudes.

So, in terms of changing stammering, if we believe this view we would embark on getting a person who stammers to feel differently about themselves, reduce any negative emotions associated with speaking, increase self-esteem and so on.

However, there was an opposing school of thought which proposed that the actual behaviour was the key. The principle behind this notion was congruence, consistency, lack of dissonance. In simpler terms this means that a person prefers to think and act in the same way. One researcher stated quite categorically that an individual infers their attitudes from what they observe themselves doing.

So, in stammering therapy, if we believe this view we would recommend that someone who stammers should experience changes in their speech before they are able to feel differently about themselves as a communicator.

All of this seems rather confusing, doesn't it? Let us fan the flames of confusion still further with a personal example. One of us learnt to swim quite late. It was around the age of 11 and swimming was never a source of real enjoyment. Some years later, while swimming alone in a lake, she briefly got out of her depth, panicked and gave herself a nasty shock before making it to the safety of dry land. From that time, until her early twenties, she avoided swimming on her own and certainly did not venture out of her depth.

It seems that an experience of a behaviour (panic in the water) brought about a change in attitude to water and swimming that subsequently meant a change in behaviour (she avoided swimming).

In later years, she was encouraged by a number of other people to improve her proficiency and work on confidence in the water. However, significant change was not brought about until she became a parent. When she realized that other people, especially her own children, could be affected by her own attitude and behaviour in water and also that her interaction with them might be compromised (that is, that she would not go swimming with them), she decided something had to change. She experienced a need to cope better. As a result, she enrolled for 'improvers' lessons (her 'therapy'?) and changed her behaviour. In subsequent years, she has been able to experience some fun times in the water with her children and now chooses to go swimming on her own for pleasure.

This example serves to illustrate that there is a link between behaviour and attitudes, each appearing to affect the other. However, this is all rather too simplistic. Instead of a linear relationship – that is, work on one and the other will change as a result – the reality is more involved. Our experience would suggest that there is a complicated interaction between attitude and behaviour, with neither one being solely dependent on the other for change. Attitude and behaviour work together, like cogs in a machine, to effect change.

As to which one starts first, we do not think that there is a cut and dried answer there either. It may be that for certain people attitude is the greater force for change and for others experiencing differences in behaviour drives them on. We have certainly met these differences in clinic. There are those people who need to experience more fluency before they can begin to feel differently about themselves, while others adopt a more thoughtful approach, talking and thinking things through before trying out new ways of behaving. Perhaps not only is it different for different people, but maybe it is also different for one person at different times. In the swimming example, perhaps there was a change in behaviour as a result of a shift in attitude when the children were born because attitudes were more susceptible to change at that time. Perhaps now given the same situation it could be that existing behaviours would be more likely to change and just going swimming on a regular basis would change the feeling about it. It may also depend on what and when we wish to change. In some instances it could be more conducive to lasting change to work on feeling differently and in others it could be more appropriate to try things out straight away.

Sometimes in clinic we have an idea about what will be the best approach to take, but a lot of the time we ask people to experiment and see what works best for them.

A theory of change

As we have seen, there are many theories about how people change, but we would like to tell you about one in particular which seems to us to make a lot of sense for those who stammer.

Two American clinical psychologists, J. O. Prochaska and C. C. DiClemente, have suggested an interesting way of looking at how people make changes in their lives. They started their research by considering the changes that are made without therapy and then at how this could be applied to change made during therapy. They came up with three important areas of change:

- 'The how' (processes).
- 'The what' (levels).
- 'The when' (stages).

We want to discuss briefly the stages of change and try to relate these to stammering. If you wish to read more of their work, we suggest you get hold of their book, *Changing for Good*, written with J. C. Norcross (further details are given in the Further reading section). Some of their work is very academic and requires considerable background knowledge of psychology and psychotherapy, but this book is user-friendly.

Through their research, Prochaska, Norcross and DiClemente discovered six stages in the change process, which are as follows.

Precontemplation

In this stage a person does not wish to change and, indeed, will resist changing. There may be a number of reasons for this. They may not think that they have a problem that needs to be changed. Perhaps they know they have a problem but feel they have no chance of changing it and so have given up hope of so doing. Those around them, however, may see things very differently and try to put pressure on the person to 'do something about it'.

We do not see many people who we feel are at this stage, although we have seen a few. One such was Bob who had given up so much that he allowed everyone else to do his talking for him, only speaking a little with his family and very close friends at home. He came to therapy because his parents were desperate to get help for him but he was much too frightened even to begin to try out any new ways of behaving. Then there was Judith. Her boss felt she would benefit from speech therapy, but she was actually quite well adjusted to her stammer and did not feel the effort involved in changing would make enough difference in her life for it to be worth while.

If you are a precontemplator, you will only be reading this book to please someone else or convince yourself or another person that change is not possible or desirable. It is more likely that someone close to you has obtained this book for you.

Contemplation

The contemplator believes they have a problem and are thinking about change. They are unsure, though, and fear both changing and staying the same. They are not yet ready to commit themselves but may spend time finding out about the problem and its treatment. We get many contemplators arriving at our doors and we need to spend time helping them explore the pros and cons of changing before we launch them into action.

Bashir was a contemplator. He could see that confronting his stammer would allow him to open new horizons in his life but also that it would be a difficult and scary task and he might fail.

If you are a contemplator reading this book, you are genuinely trying to find out what is on offer and want to consider the advantages and disadvantages of various ideas. You want to weigh up all the factors before committing yourself.

Preparation

A person in preparation has made the decision to change. They plan to start making the changes very soon and may have already experimented with some small ones. It is a time of resolution and planning.

Josh came to us at this stage. He was not without doubts, but was beginning to make some differences in his life. He talked to his boss about coming to therapy and started to try speaking at a slower rate.

As someone who is in this stage reading this book, you are probably using it to convince yourself of the sense of your decision to do something positive.

Action

This is where the change actually happens – it is a doing stage. The person is taking responsibility for their life.

Paula is currently at this stage. She is attempting feared words, talking to others openly about stammering and using the easy onset technique for some difficult words.

As a reader and an action taker, you are probably using this book to find some practical ideas.

Maintenance

The maintainer has made the desired changes but still needs to work at keeping them going and making sure they become established. They have a 'toolbox' of practical things that they can do to ensure that changes they have made are permanent.

For Geoff, these included voluntarily stammering when he felt anxious, remembering to use block modification techniques and taking on new speaking challenges.

If you are a maintainer, you may be reading this book to get some more ideas to ensure you do not slip back into your old ways or, perhaps, to refresh your memory about one or two techniques that need to be brushed up.

Termination

The terminator does not fear any relapse. They are sure that they will not return to their old behaviour. We tend to think that people who stammer rarely reach this stage but, rather, remain lifetime maintainers.

The process of change: how do you do it?

From working with adults who stammer, it seems that there is no one answer to the problem, no one thing that everyone can do which will bring about success. So, in therapy, the therapist has to present a menu of different options from which individuals can choose and find one which works best for them. We will therefore now consider a few principles of change.

Experimenting with change

One of the first things we ask a person to do is to see what happens when they change something minor in their lives, something that doesn't really matter to them. It may be they change something about their appearance. For example, Adrian chose to wear patterned socks after a lifetime of wearing only blue and black pairs. It could be a change related to a routine, such as the route taken to work, the daily newspaper read, the type of sandwiches eaten for lunch or something like that. Many people are surprised at being asked to make such changes as part of speech therapy and you can imagine the conversations people must have: 'What did you do in therapy today, dear?', 'Oh, they got me to change my socks'! On the face of it it does seem a bit odd, but there is a point to it. By experimenting with change a person can see the effect it has. It often proves to be more difficult than they imagined and they can slip easily into old patterns, familiar routines. Alternatively, they may enjoy the experience and realize that they are free to choose to act in different ways rather than follow the same old routine.

Experimenting with change also provides people with an opportunity to watch how change can affect those close to them. They can see if others are curious or threatened or appreciate the effort involved.

All this can give vital clues as to how to manage more important speech changes later on. For example, how small the steps should be, which situations would be safe to start with, which people could be involved from the beginning and so on.

Loosening

Experimenting with change also begins a phase called *loosening*, which is a term used in personal construct psychology (Kelly, 1991). Essentially, it refers to a 'freeing' of the system of constructs which a person applies to their way of living and their relationships. A 'tight' system of constructs looks like a tangled ball of wool with each of the constructs connected in some way to several of the others.

In this type of system, change is more difficult to achieve because changing one aspect will have a knock-on effect on the rest. You cannot pull one strand of wool from the ball without it affecting the whole mesh. The system needs to 'loosen' to enable change to take place.

This loosening also seems to be important for maintaining change. Some research one of us did analysed the differences in personal construct terms between good maintainers (that is, people who had managed to maintain speech-controlling techniques over a two-year period) and poor maintainers (those who were less successful). When the best maintainer in the group was compared with the poorest maintainer, it was found that one of the crucial differences was that the good maintainer was able to keep his system of constructs loose for a longer period of time than was the poor maintainer. So, perhaps the lesson here is that it is a good idea to keep experimenting with change, trying different things out for a week or two to see the effect and to find out how it feels.

Take small steps

If as non-swimmer you jump into a swimming pool at the deep end, the likelihood is that you will flounder. If, however, you enter the pool from the shallow end and learn how to swim in stages, you are more likely to cope. The same principles apply to managing change. It seems that, for most people, working in small steps works best. Each person needs to construct their own pool or hierarchy of difficulty, with a number of 'shallow', low-level situations, progressing through to the deep level of difficulty. Each level or stage needs to be tried out a number of times until the person feels confident and safe. Once is not enough. Thus, we build on success, rather than go in at the deep end right at the beginning and give up because it is too hard.

People also need to keep taking risks. They need to constantly move forwards. It would be easy to stay in the shallow end forever, where it is safe and comfortable, but if you want to be able to dive in, you have got to take the risk of moving up the pool. It's scary, but the fear does decrease as you find you can take the steps in between and your confidence develops.

Be positive

Emphasize the positive. Perhaps our culture is particularly prone to focusing on the negative. You can hear it all the time – 'Hey, you did really well there!', 'Oh, it was nothing. Just good luck.'; 'You look nice today.',

'This old thing, I've had it for years.' How can we expect to value ourselves and our achievements if we throw away this type of acknowledgement?

Similarly in our self-talk – that is, the speech that goes on in our head – we need to be registering the positive things in our lives. We must learn from situations that go right and not focus on the problems all the time. One way to do this, which has helped some people, is to have a 'positive diary'. This is simply a diary in which you record the good things that have happened or the ways in which problems or difficult situations were overcome. One woman who stammered, Dawn, took this a stage further and had what she called her 'jewels'. These were events or good times (actually, she never did tell us exactly what they were!), memories of speaking and other situations which had gone really well. These 'jewels' were brought out and recalled in darker times and they helped her keep a more positive perspective.

Another way of making sure the positive changes stick is to employ reward systems. There are a couple of techniques for rewarding positive events, which are as follows:

- *Covert management* The private words of congratulation that you can tell yourself immediately after something good has happened. These are similar to little pats on the back, which everyone needs if they are to develop positive feelings about themselves.
- *Contracts* Informal and formal contracts are often used in programmes working on change. For example, 'If I use my speech technique every day for a week, I'm going to treat myself to a curry.' Obviously the reward has to be something you would regard as a reward and not another task. You have to be very honest with yourself, too, when entering such a contract, otherwise it will not work. It may be useful to tie the reward in with the stages of the hierarchy and reward each level or stage achieved in some positive way.

Involve other people

As we discussed earlier, other people can be upset by change in those they are close to and you may need to involve them or, at the very least, provide them with some explanation for what is going on. In therapy, we have involved other people in a variety of ways.

Partners and carers can be useful observers or monitors of behaviour. John, for example, was not sure whether he had successfully cut out the amount of fillers he used in his speech. He asked his brother, with whom he had a conversation at least once a day, to give him some objective feedback and he found this was useful in helping him identify those fillers he still needed to work on. Partners and other family members can also be a help when trying out new things. It can be 'safer' to try out new behaviours in a non-threatening environment before trying it in more stressful surroundings.

Also, it can be helpful to work on a more open approach with close friends and relations. Martin talked to his wife Glenda about the difficulty he was having asking for his fare on the bus. It did not change the situation, but just knowing that someone else knew was helpful. Having a shoulder to cry on and someone to moan to when things are tough can make all the difference. Other people have talked to their significant others about stammering itself – how it feels to stammer, what it makes them feel when they do it and also asked how it is perceived from a listener's perspective.

Obviously the British Stammering Association, with its self-help groups and phonelink scheme, is a very useful source of outside support. People feel immense relief and derive great comfort from knowing that they are not the only ones in the world who are experiencing stammering problems. Talking about problems encountered in particular situations and learning how others have coped or overcome them is a great resource to be able to use.

Prepare for relapse

Finally, you need to prepare for the bad times. It is an unhappy fact of life that you cannot rely on your situation remaining constant. In fact, there is a theory that the only constant thing in life is change! You should therefore expect and prepare for more rough water in the pool, some troubled times. You can use some of the things we have talked about to help you cope at these times:

- talking to others, enlisting their support, learning how they managed;
- reading your positive diary to keep a clearer perspective – 'It's like this now, but things will be better. Remember how I coped with X' – and use the diary to find out what your strengths are and work on those, use them to your advantage;
- getting out your 'jewels', like Dawn.

In addition to these ideas, in Leeds we ask our clients to prepare their own 'toolbox', which is a number of strategies they have for coping. These can be emotional and behavioural tools – things they do and things they try to feel (we will discuss more of these ideas in a later chapter in the book).

We also suggest that people who come to us use us, their therapists, as a source of support. We often recommend a booster session, a telephone call, a letter – anything that helps and we, of course, would respond.

Summary

In this chapter we have looked at the general principles of change, what might affect how successful a person is in altering an aspect of their behaviour and the factors that could conspire against them. We have discussed a particular theory of change and applied it to stammering. Finally, we have suggested some general things to try if you yourself are ready for action.

5

How can I help myself?

Having explored some of the issues concerning the process of change, we are almost (but not quite!) ready to look at the practical aspects – what you can actually do to change. We will be discussing and describing practical techniques you can employ in the next chapter. We understand that you could now be feeling rather impatient and tempted to skip this chapter, especially as learning about the techniques may well be your main reason for reading this book. However, we ask you to bear with us a little longer before we get to these. In this chapter we will be asking you to do some preparation for the changes you may be making to your speech. Without this preparation it is likely that any changes you make will be short-lived.

So, first we want to ask you to consider how you would like to be and also what you might be prepared to settle for if your picture seems unrealistic or unobtainable. Let's explain that a bit more. Many people who stammer have as their ideal completely fluent speech. Probably this ideal is actually more fluent than the speech of so-called fluent speakers – that is, there are no hesitations, revisions, repetitions, stumblings over words and so on. *Completely* fluent speech is, in fact, almost a myth. It just doesn't happen. We suggest you watch people talking in ordinary conversations or on a discussion programme on the television to see the truth of this. Indeed, total fluency is probably not even desirable, for if we spoke in this way we would seem more like computers than people. If we are to be realistic, it is also highly unlikely that the speech of an adult who stammers will change to become like that of a person who does not stammer, however much time and effort they put into trying to make it so. They will always stammer to some extent, for example, in difficult situations or with people who make them feel ill at ease. They will always need to carry their 'toolbox' around with them so that they can carry out 'servicing' work or 'running repairs'.

Think about your own speech for a few minutes. Imagine a line with 0 at one end and 10 at the other. The 0 represents your speech at its very worst, while 10 represents your ideal speech. Now think of where you would put your average, everyday way of speaking and make a mark on the line. Next, think of the speech you would settle for and make a mark on the line at the number which best represents this. See our example opposite.

	X	X						X		X
0	1	2	3	4	5	6	7	8	9	10
worst		speech						speech		ideal
speech		now						I would		speech
								settle for		

Think some more about your speech as it is now. Write down all you know about it. Perhaps write a stammering manual, as Bryan and Diane did in Chapter 2.

Now think about the sort of speech you would settle for. How would that be? What would the person with that speech be like? How would they come across? What would they do, how would they act, what would they say? How would they start a conversation, introduce themselves, express their ideas and feelings, ask and answer questions, ask for favours, apologize, complain, end conversations and so on? Try to get a picture of this person.

Next, look at where you are currently on the scale. Say, as in our example, you are at number 2 and you would settle for number 8. Let's take one step at a time. How might you move to number 3? What is someone at number 3 like? What would you have to do to get there? How would you do all those things we mentioned in the last paragraph? If , for example, at number 2, you enter a room with your eyes fixed on the floor and without smiling, would number 3 entail trying, perhaps, to look up and smile just once? If, at number 2, you avoid all mention of your speech, might number 3 include telling just one other person about it? Think of as many differences as possible and experiment with making changes. Do not try to go to number 8 in one go, or even to 4 or 5. Just move slowly, taking one step at a time. Go gradually up the scale and take time to consolidate any progress you make.

This kind of exercise is not easy to do alone and can be quite distressing if you do not have support. We suggest you talk about it with someone close to you or consult a speech and language therapist who is trained in this kind of work, which is known as *solution-focused brief therapy*.

Having looked at what you are changing and what you want to change to, let's start to think about *how* you might change. We'll begin with some basic principles.

Confronting negative thoughts

Consider what are known as 'automatic negative thoughts' – those thoughts which have a habit of popping into your mind and influencing how you feel and act. Let's take some examples. When Amar stammers he thinks, 'I'm not as good as other people.' For John it's, 'People only see my stammer when they see me.' Susie thinks, 'I've no chance of making a good impression if I stammer.' These ways of thinking are often far from true, but thinking like this makes them seem real. Amar believes he is not as good as others and so he acts in an inferior way, almost to prove to himself that this is the case. What might he do instead? With a lot of hard work, he can learn to recognize what he is doing, confront it and alter it. He may catch himself thinking he is inferior, but say to himself, 'That's not true. I have a stammer, but I am still just as good as the next person. I have the right to express my opinions like anyone else.'

John could catch hold of his faulty thinking about how others see him. He can test it by observing people and seeing how they actually react – do they *all* seem embarrassed, anxious to finish the conversation and so on? Being more open about his stammer will put others at ease and he might even check out with people how difficult the stammer makes it to talk to him.

Susie can look at how a good impression is made – is fluent speech the only factor? What about non-verbal communication (eye contact, facial expression, gestures and so on)? How about knowing the facts, being assertive, listening well and so on? By recognizing the way in which our thinking affects our feelings and behaviour, we begin to change all three areas.

Changing feelings about stammering

In Chapter 3 we looked at how stammering develops and begins to be perceived as something you are, not just something you do. This section is about how that can change, so that much of the negative emotion associated with stammering reduces and it becomes less of a burden to carry around with you. Let's start by looking at some of these feelings about stammering commonly felt by people who stammer.

- *Fear* It is fear which fuels avoidance, fear of making a fool of yourself, of never being able to say the target word, drawing attention to yourself, feeling and being different. You are probably able to name many other fears, too. Fear can stop you doing and saying things. It can also make stammering worse by increasing tension. You reduce your fear when you begin to approach the things you fear and test out the reality. We will be looking at how to do this later in the chapter.
- *Embarrassment* If this is something you experience when you stammer, it may help to take a look at what it is you are embarrassed about. Is it that you think stammering makes you look foolish or different? Is it because

you feel your listener is embarrassed and you therefore react in a similar way? Why do you think you react in this way? How does your embarrassment affect your stammer and the effectiveness of your communication with your listener? If you can learn to stammer more openly and pay more regard to the content of your speech rather than attending purely to the fluency, you are likely to find that this feeling reduces. As one of our clients, Diane, says, 'If I didn't have the fear, I would only have a very slight problem.'

- *Shame* People who stammer often feel an enormous sense of shame. If this is so for you, you may react as though stammering is something you do deliberately which you should be able to stop at will. Accepting the stammer and not feeling a need to apologize for it can go a long way towards helping you reduce these feelings.

- *Anger* Anger is often apparent in people who stammer. It may be directed at other people, such as those who react badly or don't seem to understand what you are going through. One way of dealing with this kind of reaction is to view these people not just as merely insensitive, but as in need of education. They do not know what it is like to have a stammer (why should they?), but you might be able to explain it to them so that they can react more appropriately. A response to an impatient listener, such as, 'Please bear with me, I have a stammer and need more time to explain', can show people, quite assertively and effectively, a more appropriate way of responding. People often turn anger in on themselves. It can arise out of frustration at not feeling able to do the things they want to. Facing the difficulties and using problem-solving techniques to find alternative ways of dealing with them often reduces this kind of anger.

- *Helplessness* Many people who stammer feel they have no control and are unable to help themselves. They may even give up, believing the battle is just too great. If this is the case for you, then hopefully this book will give you a feeling of control and the knowledge that there are always things you can do. However, there may well be times when things just seem to get on top of you. When this happens and you feel unable to cope, it can help just to accept that you are going through a bad patch, to stay with it for a while, reduce the demands and look after yourself in preparation for the next step forward in tackling your stammer.

This list of negative emotions is far from exhaustive. Think about which others you experience. Look at the ways in which you may be able to start to turn them around.

Accepting the stammer

It may seem that you have no choice *but* to accept the stammer. It is there after all and it must seem as though you cannot deny that. Ask yourself, however, why, if you accept it, do you try to hide it? Sheehan, an American speech and language therapist associated with therapy aimed at reducing avoidance, believed that truly accepting the stammer was the key to change. Once a person accepts that they stammer, they stop running away from and hiding it. They no longer have to struggle and the physical and mental tension in the stammer reduces. They do not have to scan what they are saying in order to find 'easy' words to use. They do not choose activities or friends according to the speaking demands they place on them. They become more spontaneous, more relaxed and at ease with themselves as being someone who stammers but is not afraid to show it. They care more about saying the things they want to than about whether or not they can say them fluently.

If you stammer, ask yourself is it important to you to be fluent and, if so, why? What can you *not* do with a stammer that you could do if you did not stammer? Undeniably, fluency could make things easier, but does the stammer actually *prevent* you from doing anything at all? One of our clients told us that there were situations when he *had* to be fluent, but when he took some time to consider this belief he realized that, while fluency was preferable, it was certainly not essential in any aspect of his life. Try answering this question, posed by Peter Smith, a founder member of the Leeds self-help group: 'What do you lose when you run away from your stammer? We all know that if we ran away from our mortgage, we'd lose our home; if we ran away from our career, we'd lose our job, and if we ran away from our family, we'd lose them, too. All these things are unthinkable, but, of course, we run away from our stammers. But what do we lose when we do run away from our stammers?'

Being open about stammering

Being open about stammering ties in closely with acceptance. Being open means you are not afraid to talk about the stammer and the feelings connected with it. This may, for example, involve telling others that you stammer, go to speech and language therapy sessions and find some situations difficult to talk in or some words harder than others to say. It can also involve talking about stammering as and when it occurs. For example, saying, 'That was a difficult word for me to say', 'I always seem to stammer on that word', 'Words starting with an "m" cause me a lot of problems.' Talking about the covert aspects is also important. For example, you might say, 'I meant to say "coffee" not "tea", but I knew I would stammer, so I changed the word', 'I find talking in groups really difficult because of my stammer', 'Because I have a stammer I often don't feel as good as other people.' Obviously, some of these 'confessions' are more suitable to be used with people you know you can trust, but others can be used more widely.

Once you start telling people that you stammer, you will probably be surprised at the reactions you get. The majority of these will be positive. We have found that people are very interested in stammering. Often when we meet new people and they ask what we do for a living, we are bombarded with questions – 'What causes stammering?', 'What happens in therapy?', 'What should I do when I talk to someone who stammers?' and so on. It seems to be a fascinating subject to many people. Remember that others do not attach the emotion to stammering that you do and they do not view it in your negative way. If you give people the opportunity, most will want to hear what you have to say and ask you questions. Some, of course, will be fairly neutral in their responses and, very occasionally, you might come across someone who is negative. If this happens, it is important to try to put the incident behind you as quickly as possible and not to accept any blame for it. After all, it is not your fault.

When you talk to people, don't just tell them the facts, let them know about the feelings, too. Educate them about the hidden side of stammering that you are trying to bring into the open. You might see your role as that of an educator, letting people know some more about stammering and helping them respond more appropriately to you and to others they meet who stammer. The first person you inform will probably be the hardest for you, but after the first two or three, the task will start to become easier. You will begin to feel as if you have shed some of the burden of stammering instead of carrying it around with you all the time. It will start to feel less shameful to stammer. In addition, your listener will find it easier to talk to you. What often happens when you are not open is something along the lines of the following. You speak and stammer, you pretend not to have stammered, your listener pretends not to have noticed, so the conversation continues with both of you aware that you are stammering but both hiding your awareness from each other. When you give the listener 'permission' to notice by talking about the stammer, however, you both relax and the stammer seems less significant. You can then really listen to *what* each other is saying rather than *how* they are saying it and without the stammer being an unspoken demon coming between you.

Reducing your avoidance

In Chapter 2 we looked at five levels of avoidance – word, situation, feeling, relationship and self. A very important part of changing your stammer is reducing your avoidance in all these areas. However, a word of warning! You will probably have used avoidance as a way of coping and of hiding your stammer for many years. If you suddenly throw caution to the wind and decide to eliminate avoidance at a stroke, your overt stammer is likely to become much more severe. The difficulty you will face in trying to cope with this may force you back into avoiding instantly and make you less likely to try again. For this reason, we suggest that you approach avoidance reduction with some caution. Do not try to say and do all you want to at once, but, rather, work at it gradually, using a step-by-step approach.

The first step is understanding just what sorts of avoidances you use. One way of doing this is to record them over a period of time – perhaps during different kinds of conversations, for a particular length of time, with different people and so on. Notice whether or not your avoidances show any patterns. Do they, for example, occur when you are in a group rather than with individuals, on the phone, with those in authority?

You could also enlist the help of someone you trust and ask them to point out if they think you have avoided saying a particular word or been quiet when a topic you know a lot about is being discussed. Sometimes avoidance behaviours become almost second nature and are carried out without you being consciously aware of them. It can take someone else to bring them to your notice. Ask yourself what it is about situations which make it preferable to avoid rather than say the things you want to. What do you imagine would happen if you did say what you wanted? Have you ever tested this theory out?

Once you understand a little more about the nature of your avoidance behaviours you are ready to start working on them. Let us take them one by one.

Word avoidance

Remember that this takes a variety of forms, including substitution of one word for another, pretending not to know a word, talking in an accent and postponing a word by going round the houses before saying it. One technique you can use to reduce this kind of avoidance is honesty! Own up to what you have done or were tempted to do. Say something along the lines of 'I meant to say X but it's difficult for me to say and so I said Y instead.' If this proves too difficult, you could make it easier by just saying 'I meant to say X not Y.'

If you pretend to forget the word, you could 'remember' it or just look as if you are changing your mind. For example, you could say, 'I think I'd prefer tea to coffee if it's not too late to change my mind.' If there are specific words which you always avoid, you might ask a 'significant other' to ask you a question for you to reply to using that word. This exercise should be repeated over and over until your dread of the word goes. We remember using this exercise with a teenager who felt he could not answer the register because his teacher's name was difficult to say. We decided that he would stop calling his Mother 'Mum' for a while and refer to her as 'Mrs Shufflebottom'! It did the trick – he became confident in answering the register (and his Mother was relieved to drop her new title!).

Another useful strategy is to set yourself avoidance 'targets'. You may, for example, only allow yourself a set number of avoidances each day. When you have had your 'ration', you have to say any other difficult words. Don't be too hard on yourself at first, but gradually increase the difficulty of the task as you increase in confidence. An alternative could be to choose difficult words which you have to bring into a conversation.

Situation avoidance

Identifying those factors which make you more likely to avoid a particular situation is an important first step in modifying this kind of avoidance. Try to find out why you avoid one situation and not another. Is it because of the numbers or types of people involved – large groups or people in authority, for example? Is it more to do with the words you have to say, your name, address, a specific bus fare and so on? Could it be because you experienced a particularly difficult stammering episode in a similar situation before and the emotion keeps coming back to you when you are in that situation again?

Understanding the reasons behind the difficulty can help you as you start to face it. It can help you to break down your task into manageable components. Let's look at an example of this.

Colin

Colin avoids talking in groups. In fact, his friends have stopped asking him to go to the pub with them because they get fed up with hearing his excuses for not coming and think that he doesn't enjoy their company. Colin chooses to let them think this, although in reality he would love to take them up on their offer. For Colin, however, refusing them is preferable to letting them see him stammer severely. He is sure this would happen if he did go out with them.

So, what can Colin do? It seems like a catch-22 situation. If he stays at home, he misses out on some of his friendships and risks his friends thinking all manner of things about him. If he does go out with them, he feels they will find out his guilty secret and think badly of him. However, is this really the case?

There are other possibilities he has not considered. For example, he may not stammer or his stammer will not be as severe in this situation as he fears. If he does stammer, his friends may not see things in the same way as Colin fears. Perhaps they will not notice the stammer anywhere near as much as he thinks. If they do notice, their response could be understanding and caring. Maybe they will not see stammering in the same negative way that Colin does. Has Colin ever considered the possibility that they care far more about Colin's company than about whether or not he stammers?

Colin can use these alternative ways of thinking to help himself take the plunge and enter the dreaded situation. He might prepare for it in a number of ways. He could tell one of his closest friends in the group about his fears and see what his reaction is. He could go to the pub but start off by doing more listening than speaking. He could use voluntary stammering (see Chapter 6) so that people hear his stammer in control before they hear it out of control and he can look at them in order to ascertain their reaction. He can ask himself if he really wants to let his stammer control important aspects of his life or if he wants to regain some of the control he has relinquished.

Feeling avoidance

Again, you need to ask yourself what factors are involved in any feeling avoidance you do. Let us take some examples from our clincal experience and see how our clients have gone about reducing this kind of avoidance.

Bernard did not like to apologize. For him, it felt like a sign of weakness when his stammer already made him feel inferior. He needed to examine the logic of such a belief. Once he discovered that apologizing was actually an act of assertiveness, he was able to do more of it and eventually feel more comfortable and in control.

Paul found it hard to show anger as it disrupted his fluency. He thus bottled up these feelings and they had the habit of 'spilling over' at inappropriate times. Once he started to let his feelings out as soon as he felt them, he found that he did not stammer as much as he feared and those around him preferred to know where they were with him.

Relationship avoidance

For some people, one of the factors in relationship avoidance is related to lack of experience. Do you hold back from meeting others because of your concern about speaking? Maybe you wait for others to approach you rather than make the first move. This unfamiliarity in areas such as greetings, partings, continuing conversations, turntaking and so on leads to lack of confidence. This reinforces the vicious circle of avoidance, lack of confidence, more avoidance, more lack of confidence and so on. Sometimes people need to learn these skills (perhaps on a confidence-building, social and communication skills or assertiveness course, either through speech and language therapy or further education). Others have the skills in some areas of their life but need to take the plunge and extend them into new areas and discover that people are generally more interested in the person and what they have to say, than they are in the fluency of the person's delivery. Try to relate this to yourself.

Avoidance of your self with a stammer

This is the big one! If you remember from Chapter 2, it is about accepting that you stammer and giving up the struggle continually to present yourself as fluent. There is no easy way to do this and it can be a long and difficult task. Essentially, the activities outlined in this chapter are all about reducing this kind of avoidance. It will not go overnight, but with determination, support and encouragement you can learn to feel differently.

Being the real you

Suppose you woke up tomorrow morning and, during the night, a miracle had happened and your stammer had disappeared. As you were asleep when the miracle happened you are not aware of what has transpired. Ask yourself how you would find out. The answer you give will be an individual one.

You may think you would know before you spoke. This would perhaps be because you had a feeling inside that things were different or a lack of doom and gloom about the day ahead, an optimism, a belief that you could face whatever the day brought. It may be that you would not find out until you first spoke. It could be someone else who noticed first – your partner, housemate, child or parent. How might your day progress? What would you do or say that would be different? How would you feel? How would others see you? How would you react to them and they react to you? Might you, for example, be more assertive, say the things you really want to rather than hope things go your way by chance? Could it be that you would smile more, keep better eye contact, use more gestures, stop fidgeting? Might you find yourself concentrating on your listener and on what they are telling you through their non-verbal and verbal communication rather than worrying about what they are going to say next and whether or not you can say it fluently? Instead of scanning ahead for difficult words, would you say exactly what you wanted?

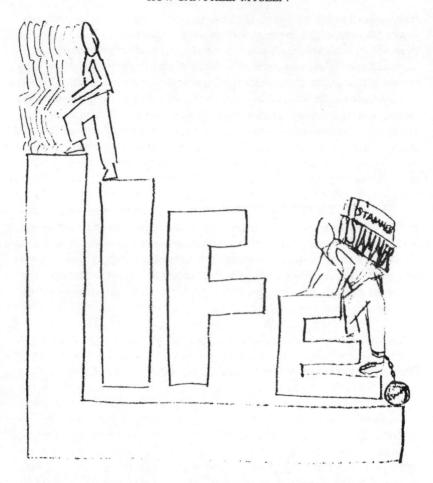

Figure 2 A client's picture of their stammer

As you start to think about how you would be after the miracle, ask yourself if you might be able to learn something from your thoughts which would help you to live the miracle *now*. This is what we mean when we say 'be the real you'. Stammering is so often like a prison, many of the bars having been created by the person who stammers, until they are so close together that escape seems impossible. Because they fear stammering and others' reactions to it, people who stammer often put up barriers, trying to act as though they are fluent and in this way they change from being the person

68

they really are. This has become clear to us over the years in a number of ways. Often it is through things we hear our clients say, such as 'People think I am shy, but really I am an extrovert inside', 'I come across as ignorant, but actually I know a lot about the subject, I just can't say it', 'I'm often described as nervous, but I am really quite a confident person.' Another way we have discovered this facet of stammering is by using artwork. We ask the person who stammers to draw a picture of their stammer (see Figure 2). Very often there is an aspect of imprisonment in their art – sometimes represented by bars, high walls, dead ends, barriers to overcome and so on.

Our work involves helping people find ways to pull down the walls or remove the bars – not all at once but one at a time. One way in which we try to do this is to help our clients test out the reality of behaving as they would like to, to be themselves instead of acting as if they were fluent. This means taking risks – saying the words you want to, not the ones that mean something slightly different but that you can say fluently, speaking to someone with whom you want to have a conversation, rather than hoping that they will initiate the conversation, looking for a job you want to do rather than choosing a job because the speaking demands are minimal, using the phone to book a ticket rather than travelling to somewhere where you can book face to face. The list is endless, but all the things on your own list should involve being the person you really are rather than the person you may currently be letting your stammer dictate that you are. Don't wait for the miracle to happen, be your own miracle worker!

6
Practical ideas

In this chapter we will look at some practical skills and techniques. Some of the ideas are fairly straightforward and can be put into practice without therapy. To implement others you will need guidance. It is important when considering the use of techniques to be aware that no two people who stammer are the same and an approach which helps one may not be helpful to another. We would also ask you always to keep in mind the principles we outlined in the last chapter. Doing this should ensure that any techniques you employ will increase both your confidence and your control over your speech, not encourage you to hide and avoid your stammer.

These ideas are not written in a specific order, nor according to importance, but, rather, we have tried to group ideas according to themes. Thus, for example, non-verbal techniques are close to each other, as are speech control techniques.

Ideally, the techniques are best used under the direction of a speech and language therapist specializing in dysfluency. This is because they can discuss those that are most useful for you, bearing in mind any previous therapy you may have had and what it is you wish to achieve.

You will see that we have included comments by people who stammer at the ends of the sections. We hope you will find these a useful extra something that will help you decide if that particular technique could be of use to you.

Speed of speech and pausing

If you have stammered all your life, we expect you will have lost track of the number of times well-intentioned people have told you to 'slow down', as if this would be the answer to all your problems. If only it were as simple as that! Slowing down alone is not the answer to stammering, but it can help some people.

If you slow down, you give yourself more time to speak, you feel more in control, can analyse what is happening in your speech and have time to consider other techniques you might apply. There are also advantages to your listener. You will probably be easier to listen to, seem less flustered about speaking and appear more confident and controlled.

Perhaps we should first consider why people who stammer sometimes speak more quickly than others and whether you are yourself a fast speaker.

In the general population, people speak at a variety of speeds. The so-called 'normal' rate of speech is around 110–170 words per minute (or 150–250 syllables per minute) and it can be difficult for a listener to take in what is being said if the rate is too far either side of this norm.

If you are unsure of your own speech rate, you could tape record yourself in a number of situations – reading, talking by yourself, talking to one other person and talking in a group, for example. Then, isolate one minute's talking from each of these situations and count the number of words or syllables to see what your speech rate is. If this seems rather too complicated, just listen to yourself and compare your speech rate to that of other people or ask them if they think you speak too quickly (if they do, they may well have told you so already!).

People who stammer sometimes speak too quickly because they have a sense of urgency about what they are saying, a feeling that they have to keep going to stop themselves from getting stuck, to prevent someone from interrupting them or because they fear not being able to get started again. Many people who stammer do not talk any more quickly than others. However, it seems that some speak too quickly to keep control over their speech muscles.

So, what can you do about your speed if you feel it is a problem for you? Here are a few ideas.

Learn to monitor your speech rate – if you listen to yourself carefully and implement the ideas mentioned above, you can become aware of when you are speaking too quickly. Awareness is the first step towards changing something.

Ask others to tell you if they feel you are talking too quickly for them. You will need to consider carefully who you ask to do this and how you will treat their reminders. It is no use asking someone to do this if you then ignore what they say or become annoyed with them when they have done as you asked. Think about *when* you want them to tell you (when you are alone, in company, with which people), for how long you want them to monitor you at a time (five minutes, half an hour, whenever they notice), how they will do it (a word, a sign) and how you will acknowledge their reminder (by a smile, saying 'thank you', by trying to slow down). If you do not use the prompts, the person is likely to stop giving them.

Think about the message you are trying to put across and where to pause to make the meaning most clear. Pausing serves a number of functions in reducing speech rate. It can help you slow down your overall speech rate. It is also more difficult for you to speed up after a pause, so it reduces your rate in this way, too.

Try to resist pressure to speed up when you become agitated or involved in what you are saying. We recognize that this is not an easy task but practise will help. It is a good idea to slow down other things too – the way you walk, eat, carry out routines and so on. We have found that this is the key for some people. We recall one man who realized as a result of this sort of experiment that his whole life was conducted in a rush – no wonder his speech rate reflected this same sense of urgency. Once he slowed down these other things, he found that it was easier to slow his speech and he felt much more in control.

Some comments

To me, speed control seems to be the most productive way of controlling my stammer. Not just taking time with my word pronunciations or letting my mind race ahead causing me to fall head first into one of the all-time great blocks, but slowing down certain aspects of my everyday life. For example, picking up the phone gently and calmly when it rings or writing a little slower or after being asked a question, taking a little more time to answer. I suppose it is a way of collecting my thoughts, relaxing my whole speech process and trying to maintain a good level of control over my speech.

Speed and rate control doesn't come overnight, it takes a lot of self-teaching and discipline. I suppose there will always be the odd time when I slip into my old habits, but for now I feel to be firmly in the driving seat, which in turn gives me more confidence in the complicated art of conversation.

Andrew Johnstone

While speed control cannot be a therapy on its own, because it is not dealing with other problems of stammering such as desensitization, anxiety, avoidance, fears, etc., speed is a major problem for most stammerers. They tend to speak fast and lose control of their speech. I, for one, have benefited hugely from just slowing down and controlling my speech.

Nasser Karimi

Breathing

Breathing is one of the most important mechanisms in speaking. It is breath which is the power supply to our voices, providing the fuel to make the vocal cords vibrate and thus create sound. Breath control also has an important role in sustaining the sound. If we do not breathe properly, our speech will be adversely affected.

So what is good breathing? There are two phases to the breathing cycle – breathing in (inspiration or inhalation) and breathing out (expiration or exhalation). Let us look at these in turn.

Breathing in

When we breathe in as we prepare for speech, we need to take in enough air to say a whole phrase which makes sense to the listener. If we are saying a single word, we will need very little air, but if we are speaking a long sentence, we have to be sure there is enough air for the sound to keep going. This does not mean we should say extremely long sentences without pausing for breath, but merely that we need enough air for the amount we have to say in one go. Beware, however, of taking in larger amounts of breath with a 'gasp'. Just take your time and breathe in a relaxed way, filling your lungs with air. (We are aware that some clients have been told by well-meaning others to 'stop and take a deep breath' when they start to stammer. This has resulted in the development of an abnormal pattern of breathing, which should be avoided at all costs.)

Air is taken into our lungs through our nose and/or mouth. It goes from here to the windpipe and thence to the lungs. In order for the lungs to have space to receive the air, they need to be able to expand – rather like balloons or bellows. Room for this expansion is created in two ways. The ribs move outwards and the diaphragm (a band of muscle below your ribs) moves downwards and outwards. Because of the shape of the ribcage, the area which can expand the most is at the bottom of the lungs, so this is where the most movement needs to take place to ensure efficient intake of air.

Breathing out

When we breathe out, the opposite happens. The ribs are drawn back in and the diaphragm comes to rest by returning upwards and inwards. The air comes out of the lungs, up the windpipe and out through your nose and mouth. It is this exhaled air which is used in speaking. If we have not taken in enough air, then the air we breathe out will not be sufficient to sustain the sound. We will need to take in more breaths, which can then be disruptive and may build up unnecessary tension.

If you feel your breathing is not adequately controlled, you may find it helpful to do some breathing exercises. Here are some you might try:

- Stand up or sit in an upright chair in a relaxed position. Put your hands on your lower ribs so that the fingers of your two hands just touch each other. As you breathe in, your hands move slightly apart, but your shoulders remain still and there should be very little movement in your chest (if you look in a mirror as you do this, it may help you to notice exactly what is happening).

- Breathe in at an even pace, remaining relaxed. When we speak, this phase of breathing happens quite rapidly. However, be careful not to become tense. Let the breath out slowly and see how many seconds you can keep it going. Make sure you let the air out evenly.
- Repeat the last exercise, but this time let the air out as you say the sound 's'. You should be able, with practice, to make the sound last about 20 seconds.

Some comments

This is one area in which I had to (and still do) put in quite a bit of practice, as at pre-therapy my style of breathing was atrocious. My diaphragm was almost constantly clenched, meaning that I only really breathed with my upper chest. This resulted in my taking frequent, shallow breaths which often resulted in running out of air mid-sentence. Alternatively, when I knew that I was about to speak, I would often over-breathe, taking in huge lungfuls of air which habitually led to the muscles in my chest and vocal apparatus becoming so tense as to cause instantaneous blocking.

Thankfully, I have managed to modify my way of breathing to the extent that, as far as I am aware, few of the blocks I now experience are related to the way I breathe. I have tried to retrain myself to breathe in a slower and more relaxed manner, using both chest and diaphragm in harmony. My diaphragm is rarely clenched now, which, aside from greatly aiding breathing, also feels more comfortable physically. I now try to breathe between phrases when I am speaking, which has also had impact upon my speaking rate.

Mark Birdsall

Light contacts

This term concerns the way you form the sounds of speech. Some people who stammer produce their sounds with too much tension, which results in a harsh way of talking and often makes stammering more likely. This may be apparent in most speech sounds or just some. Particularly vulnerable to this kind of attack are the plosive sounds, which are 'p', 'b', 't', 'd', 'k' and 'g'. These are made by putting together certain of the speech muscles and allowing air to build up behind the contact until air pressure forces them apart and the sound is produced. If we take the sound 'p' as an example, the lips are put together, air pressure builds up in the mouth cavity behind the lips and the pressure is then released, resulting in the 'p' sound being made.

When sounds are made with light contacts, these contacts are relaxed. Again taking 'p' as an example, the lips are 'placed' rather than 'pushed' together. The resulting sound is gentle and relaxed. If you practise, you can learn to produce sounds in this softer way. Try to notice what is happening in your mouth when you talk. Keep your lips relaxed, watch your tongue is not pressed hard against the roof of your mouth and do not let your jaws bite together as you talk. Really feel what you are doing and notice the difference between when contacts are hard and when they are soft.

As well as helping to reduce the tension in your speech and making stammering less likely, speaking in this way can also make your speaking voice sound relaxed and pleasant to listen to.

A comment

When I analyse my blocks and when I see others blocking, many of the physical difficulties of speaking which I encounter can be attributed to the use of hard contacts. The excessive muscular tension which characterizes this problem and elicits blocking is perhaps analogous to trying to force a very large square peg through a very small round hole. Although it seems that any sound can be problematical (if attacked fiercely enough), plosives and fricatives seem to lend themselves to hard contacts. This is no doubt because the articulation of these types of sounds demands a degree of tension in the vocal apparatus anyway (i.e. in the lips, tongue and so on). Having employed this technique for a while now, I find that I very often use it unconsciously. As a means to greater fluency, I have found it very beneficial. Using it also helps minimize word avoidance. If the peg doesn't fit the hole, change the hole, not the peg!

Mark Birdsall

Easy onset

Akin to light contacts is the technique of easy onset. This is used at the beginning of a sentence or after a breath or a pause. It is especially useful for people who find it difficult to get started and is a way of simplifying the speaking process.

When we speak, we use exhaled air. As we start to breathe out, we often start to make the speech sound at the same time. There is some evidence which suggests that people who stammer find this simultaneous action hard to co-ordinate. In easy onset, the two phases are separated and breathing out starts slightly before any sound is made.

We suggest you practise this technique initially on single words, starting with vowel sounds. You can then go on to practise it with easy consonant sounds and finally with plosives (see Appendix I for some lists of these words to use when you are practising). It tends to be most difficult to use this technique with the plosive sounds. You may find the 'explosive' nature of the sound becomes slightly changed as you stretch it (for example, 't' in 'too' may sound a little like 'ts').

The process we suggest you use is as follows:

1 Let out a little air, slowly and gently. We stress 'just a little' – you are only starting off the exhalation process and must be careful not to use too much air or you will run out of breath too soon. We sometimes describe this as a 'puff' of air, but this can make it sound as if it is let out forcefully, which is certainly not the case. Another way of describing it is as a silent 'h' sound – but be careful that it really is silent or your speech may sound rather strange.
2 Start to make the sound slowly and gently, slightly stretching the first sound and using a light contact as described above under Light contacts.
3 Move slowly into the next sound of the word.
4 Complete the rest of the word a little more quickly, but still hold on to the feeling of control.

Once you have practised this technique with single words, you can go on to try two-word utterances, building up to short phrases. Practise at home initially, perhaps while reading or using our word lists. Then, try the technique out 'for real', in front of someone close to you. Next, experiment with using it in other situations in which you feel at ease. It may take a while before you are ready to use the technique in conversation. We suggest that you practise it regularly first to build up your confidence and to help the technique become more automatic and natural before you try it with someone else.

For many, this technique is very valuable and an aid to feeling in control. It can be used in time as a matter of course, especially when you start speaking, which is when people often anticipate having most difficulty.

A comment

I find easy onset a useful tool. It is rather like a sport in that it improves with practice and is something you can practise at home before trying it outside. I always used to have trouble saying my name – that initial 'D' was a killer. Easy onset now enables me to say my name effectively 95 per cent of the time. This is a big improvement on 0 per cent, despair level.

I practised this at home by recording a tape of me saying 'What is your name?' in many different tones of voice and variations (e.g., 'tell me your name', 'name?', 'and your name is?', etc.), leaving spaces between each recording so that when I played it back I could practise saying the dreaded 'D' word using easy onset. It is surprising how effective this method is. From there, I went on to answering the phone with my name. This is something I still do with every incoming call. Easy onset has shown me that I do not have to glue my tongue to the roof of my mouth every time I try to say a word. I now have a choice provided by the introduction to, and constant practice of, easy onset.

Daniel Hunter

Slowed speech

This is a technique which was very popular with some therapists and clients in the late 1970s and 1980s. You may well have learnt it if you had therapy at that time. It is still used by some therapists and a number of clients find it very helpful, but it is no longer seen as the cure-all it was once thought to be.

Slowed speech consists of a number of features used as a 'package', but with differing aspects that are especially useful to particular people. Some of these are described elsewhere in this chapter, namely light contacts, which we covered earlier, controlled breathing, pausing, both covered at the beginning of this chapter, and relaxation, covered in the next section. The other features of the technique are as follows:

- *A slow rate of speech* The technique is first learnt at an exceedingly slow rate, usually about 30 syllables per minute. This speed is not intended to be used other than in the clinic or at home when practising. It allows everything about the technique to be exaggerated, so it sounds rather like an old gramophone record being played at the wrong speed! Gradually the person learns to speed up this speaking rate, so that they use a slow average rate while feeling very much in control.
- *Flow* The sounds of speech are rolled together so that the transitions between sounds and words are not jerky and there are no gaps in the person's speech, except when they are pausing. It may help to imagine the end of one word becoming the beginning of the next. An example might be 'Sunday lunch' said as 'S-u-n-d-a-y-l-u-n-c-h'.
- *Prolongation* This involves drawing out sounds in speech so that they last fractionally longer than usual. This helps to stop tension building up and keeps speech smooth and controlled. The vowel sounds (a, e, i, o and u) tend to be the easiest sounds to do this with but it is important to prolong

the other sounds (consonants), too, in order to avoid speech becoming overly rhythmical.

One of the difficulties people find in employing slowed speech comes from the fact that it needs to be used all the time in order to be effective. This means using it when speech would normally be fluent as well as when it would be stammered. It takes enormous will-power and concentration to do this and, even with lots of motivation, the technique can break down at times of stress.

Another problem we have heard people mention time and time again is that when they use slowed speech it just doesn't feel 'like them'. This problem of the person feeling their speech is alien to them is perhaps why the technique is so difficult to maintain. However, we have known a few people who have been able to use slowed speech very successfully and maintain a high level of fluency most of the time. We have to say, though, that there are far more who have learnt to use it well but have abandoned its use because of the difficulties we have outlined.

There are considerably more people who have used certain aspects or limited combinations of slowed speech to their advantage rather than taking on board the whole package. One person, for example, may find light contacts particularly helpful while, for another, flow is the key and yet another benefits from, say, prolongation and rate control. You may wish to experiment with different aspects to see which, if any, are helpful in your situation.

A comment

For a naturally quick speaker, which I am, slowed speech is a very good technique. It reduces rushing into difficult words or speaking situations and forces me to treat each sound as an equal. When a sound is approaching on which I would be afraid of blocking, slowing down my speech gives time to think out strategies to reduce the fear, relax muscles and, hopefully, glide slowly over the offending article.

It is a most natural technique and, best of all, can be made to sound 'normal' with practice. Many effective speakers talk very slowly and quietly. It makes the audience listen and the speaker has time to eradicate all the unnecessary filler words and sounds, leaving in just the important ones. I feel very much in control when speaking slowly, and self-confidence follows quickly. Different degrees of slowed speech can be used to suit the occasion. It needs considerable practice to become second nature, but it is the kind of thing which family, friends and colleagues can help with if they have the method properly explained first. In slowed speech, of course!

Mike Peace

Relaxation

Like many people who stammer, you may experience tension in your speech muscles and, perhaps, other parts of your body, too (see Chapter 2). Learning to relax can be one way of in helping you feel and speak better.

Before you try any relaxation techniques, you need to identify where the tension is occurring in your body. Is it general or specific? Be aware of areas such as your limbs, chest, stomach, neck and throat, jaws and face where tension commonly appears. Is the tension there only when you are speaking or is it apparent all the time? While the tension in your upper body will more directly affect your speech, tension in the rest of the body can also be significant as it tends to have a knock-on effect.

There are two main approaches to achieving general relaxation. One involves tensing and then letting go of tension. The second involves concentrating on sensations within your body and on increasing the relaxation by focusing on these feelings. There is a useful booklet entitled *You Can Change: A self-help guide to the management of stress* by Diane Eaglen and Debs Plummer, specialist speech and language therapists, outlining these two approaches, suggesting some exercises you can carry out, and including other techniques for stress reduction (see the Further reading section for the address to write to for a copy).

We frequently use the second of the approaches and in Appendix II we outline a relaxation routine you might want to use. It is adapted from a technique called Anxiety Control Training, devised by Snaith (1974) which also aims to find ways in which to help you control your anxiety. Note that you will need the help of someone trained in using this last technique if you want to use it in this way and if you are to find the routine helpful, you will need to practise it regularly.

As well as carrying out any specific relaxation routines, you should try to develop an awareness of when you are becoming tense. As we have seen, people often find that there are specific areas of the body where they get tense and particular times when the tension occurs. One of us, for example, gets physically very tense when driving long distances on motorways and once we realize what is happening and let the tension go, we find that our shoulders seem to drop several centimetres! Other people notice that they are clenching their fists, pulling back or tapping a foot, biting their lip, pulling at their hair and so on when they are tense.

Developing good posture can also help reduce tension. Try to sit or stand straight, but not too rigidly. Do not slouch, but maintain an erect position which facilitates good breathing. Be particularly aware of the muscles of your chest, throat and face. Aim to keep these areas especially relaxed. Research findings suggest that if these areas are continually under tension, the actual shape of the vocal tract can change, affecting speech even more.

Some comments

During my search for the magical cure for my stammer I have done a lot of relaxation exercises. I did them dutifully (as any good client should), but never really questioned their effectiveness. Then one day I was reading a stress management book which dismissed the whole ethos of relaxation by saying that the moment you came out of your self-induced state you went right back into your everyday life, your everyday stresses and, in my case, your everyday stammer. The author certainly had a point but he wasn't totally correct. He missed the vital component of relaxation. Learning how to do it is easy. Doing it is easy. Transferring those feelings to everyday situations is difficult; difficult, but not impossible. Transfer, I began to think, was the key to successful relaxation. From that day on I taught myself to transfer the way I felt during relaxation to everyday difficult speaking situations – and it worked. Now when my shoulders tense and the veins on my neck are ready to burst, I let it go . . . let it go . . . let it go . . . and by relaxing the major muscles of my body I find it does have a knock-on effect on my speech and makes me more fluent. I feel more relaxed, I certainly look more relaxed (which incidentally makes my listener feel more comfortable and relaxed) and my speech is less tense and jerky. Now if I'm asked whether or not relaxation works, I have to say 'yes', but only if it is transferred from the comfort of your own home and used as a positive tool in difficult speaking situations.

Daniel Hunter

Relaxation is beneficial to everyone. Specifically aimed at the stammerer, however, it has even more use as part of a whole strategy. It gives time out of the hubbub of a stressful life; for to relax properly one should lay down in a quiet room. It gives the opportunity to monitor physical tension or mental turmoil and to reduce their harmful effects. Problems can be put into perspective, heart rates slowed down, large and small groups of muscles can be relaxed and breathing changes from shallow, quick gasps to deep, slow breaths, using the diaphragm. It gives time to think about the stammer in a calm and analytical way, rather than pushing it to the back of the shelf in the hope that it may go away.

Done regularly, daily or twice daily, it can become automatic. It is then no longer necessary to use the quiet room in which to relax. One becomes more aware of tense hands on a steering wheel or clenched stomach or chest muscles in a meeting. If a time of anxiety occurs, any tension can be spotted and worked on. Shoulders will fall, the mouth smiles, hands lay cool and relaxed in the lap and speech may become more calm and controlled.

Mike Peace

Voluntary stammering

If you have not heard about this term before, you may wonder, as we are sure many of our clients do, if we are in our right minds when we suggest people should stammer on purpose! However, we assure you that voluntary stammering is a tried and tested approach which in the past 60 or so years has been helpful to thousands of people who stammer. It is not a technique in the usual sense as it is not aimed at making your speech better, but it is a good foundation for block modification, which we describe next.

In essence, voluntary stammering is a form of desensitization, a way of helping you to feel less sensitive about stammering. It is useful for a number of reasons:

- When you stammer deliberately, you are stammering in control – you learn that stammering does not have to be something which has a life of its own, and you are in charge of when it starts, stops and how long it lasts.
- You are letting people know that you stammer, rather than waiting to see whether they will find out, which can take away a lot of anticipated fear, and you may find this helps you enjoy conversations more.
- You can observe people's reactions to stammering – one of the features of this approach is that you look at the person as you stammer, which is a change from the usual as, so often when stammering, people avoid eye contact and therefore cannot make an objective assessment.
- You are deciding how to stammer and learning that stammering does not have to be associated with struggle – you will find this helpful if you later come to modify your actual stammering.
- Voluntary stammering is the opposite of avoidance – you are no longer hiding from your stammer, but, instead, are approaching it in a calm, controlled way.

There are two approaches to voluntary stammering. We suggest you use

81

them both. The first, *repetition*, involves repeating the first sound of a word slowly about three times. This is enough to allow others to notice the stammer but not too much to prevent you from having a go! Thus, if you were doing this on the word 'banana you would say 'b,b,b, banana'. The other approach is called *prolongation*, also known as a *slide*. This involves extending the sound to make it last a little longer. Some sounds are easier to do this with than others. For example, sounds such as 's', 'm', 'l', 'f' and all the vowel sounds (a, e, i, o and u). Other sounds – for example, 'b', 'd' and 'g' – do not lend themselves so easily to prolongation and need to be softened somewhat first. Make sure you keep your head still as you stammer. Do not nod in time to the repetitions or slide along with the prolongations! Also, bear in mind the following:

- Always look at the person with whom you are voluntarily stammering. Remember, you are not trying to hide the stammer. You are showing the person you are stammering but are in control, so you want to see their reaction.
- Your stammering should be slow and deliberate – do not try to rush through it.
- Initially, you should stammer voluntarily only on sounds or words you do not fear and on which you do not expect to stammer. For many people these will be words which do not carry much importance, such as 'the', 'and' and so on. If you tend to stammer more at the beginning of a sentence, you should not try to use the approach there. All of these factors reduce the likelihood of the voluntary stammer turning into a real one.
- Use the approach at first in situations where you do not mind stammering. You may want to practise it initially at home with someone close to you or alone as you read. When you become more experienced and more comfortable using it, you can start applying it in situations which cause you anxiety. Many people report that voluntary stammering takes away their fear of stammering in such situations. You may, or may not, want to tell people what you are doing. In our experience, some people find this helpful, while others do not. One of our clients, Gillian, told her friends and family and gained support and encouragement to stammer voluntarily – in fact, they would do it with her if she asked them. On the other hand, Philip told his wife and she found the concept impossible to understand and so did all she could to stop him using it. We therefore suggest you start off by using just one or two voluntary stammers a day in a 'safe situation'. Gradually extend the number you use and the situations in which you use them.
- Sometimes people are concerned that a voluntary stammer will turn into a

real one. In our experience, this happens far less frequently than you would imagine. If it does happen it is usually because the person is either voluntarily stammering too quickly or is stammering on a word that they fear. Should it happen, you should aim to keep calm. After all, the object of the exercise is to desensitize yourself to your stammer, and keeping calm is a good way of doing so!

Some comments

Voluntary stammering is one of the best 'tools' for any stammerer who is serious about taking control of their own speech. It serves a number of tasks in the quest for improved speech. The way it helped me was to:

● prove to myself that I could stammer openly, feel in control and actually enjoy the stammering experience;
● desensitize myself, show the listener that I have a stammer and can be in control when I do stammer, therefore reducing the dread of stammering which can be brought about by trying to conceal it;
● allow me to look at the listener and to assess their reaction to my stammer logically, without my thoughts being clouded by my fear of stammering.

So, when I voluntarily stammer, I say to myself, 'Look at me! I can look you straight in the eye, stammer and still feel in complete control!' It's a great feeling and one I would recommend.

Bryan Wood

A very confrontational technique this, which no doubt explains why many people who stammer have difficulty using it habitually. The benefits behind using it can be very difficult to grasp when you are being asked to go out into the real world and stutter *on purpose*! Applying this technique, particularly at first, forced me to break the habit of a lifetime and purposely reveal my dysfluency, albeit in a controlled and intentional way. As such, I believe that voluntary stammering can be very helpful in gradually desensitizing oneself to one's stammer. It also allowed me to stutter while at the same time feeling in complete control, something which admittedly sounds like a complete contradiction in terms! Finally, by using this technique, I discovered that, when I did stammer, people generally didn't appear all that bothered. This was quite a staggering discovery and probably something I couldn't have become aware of without using it. When I was in a true block I would get so caught up in my *own* feelings of embarrassment and foolishness that I would automatically assume that whoever was listening would also think that of me. To find out that this was rarely the case forced me to reassess many of my previous certainties about the attitudes of others towards my dysfluency.

Mark Birdsall

Block modification

Block modification is the term used for a series of techniques used to modify or change the stammer. Unlike slowed speech, which is used as a replacement for the person's normal speech (both stammered and fluent), block modification is used to change the moment of stammering only. In slowed speech, the aim is for the person to *speak* more fluently, while in block modification the person aims to *stammer* more fluently. This distinction will become clearer with further explanation.

This approach was developed by the American clinician Charles Van Riper over a period of 20 years. Incidentally, he also stammered throughout his life but learned excellent control by using his own therapy procedures. He believed that the struggle and avoidance associated with stammering were learnt behaviours which could therefore be unlearnt, resulting in easier stammering (but not fluency). Van Riper outlined four stages of therapy – identification, desensitization, modification and stabilization. We have already talked about the first two of these in Chapters 2 and 5. Here we will briefly describe the modification phase. The idea is to change the stammer, so that tension is reduced and the word can be said with greater control. It is not a simple process and if you feel it is something you would like to try, we suggest you do so with a therapist rather than just have a go by yourself.

The modification phase has three parts. These are known as cancellation (post-block modification), pull-outs (in-block modification) and pre-sets (pre-block modification). You start learning to modify the stammer *after* it has occurred, then move on to modifying it *as it* occurs and eventually *before* it occurs.

Cancellation

As its name suggests, this phase is about cancelling out a stammer which has already occurred. When you stammer, the tendency is to 'push through' the block, using varying degrees of force, in order to produce the word you want to say. The reward for pushing through comes when you finally say the word, and often you will experience some fluency with the words you say next. Essentially, cancellation stops you getting this reward and makes it less likely that you will struggle through each successive stammer.

There are several stages in cancellation. In essence, it involves learning by stages to pause after you have completed a stammered word, identifying what went wrong and made you stammer, thereby discovering a new way of saying the word more fluently.

Pull-outs

In cancellation you work on your stammer after it has happened. With pull-outs, you learn to do something about it as it is happens. You should not move on to this stage until you are able to cancel a considerable number of your stammers. There are different approaches for dealing with different types of stammers.

If you try to use pull-outs but do not achieve what you set out to do, it is important that you then cancel the stammer. In this way you still succeed in doing something positive about your stammer.

Pre-sets

This is the last stage of modification. Here you anticipate a stammer and deal with it before it occurs. As in the other stages, several processes are involved.

If you are unsuccessful at using pre-sets at any time, then you can use pull-outs. If you do not succeed with these, use cancellation. You should always aim to do something to modify the stammer to ensure a feeling of success.

A comment

I'm a big fan of block mod. It is essentially a very positive technique which endows me with many choices, not just concerning whether or not I stammer but also how I stammer. It is a graded learning process which has taken me from a situation where I constantly either hid my stammer or ran out of options and stammered wildly, to one whereby I can exert control over the way I stammer. Block mod is, however, no 'pink pill' cure. At first it is very confrontational. The first time I used cancellation I felt very foolish. It is difficult and takes time to master.

What I especially like about block mod is that you cannot fail. Failure is not an option. There are so many 'safety nets' inherent in this system that the term 'do or die' is not applicable. If I cannot manage a pre-block I try an in-block; if that is too difficult I cancel the word and if I have no success there I can go back to doing some voluntary stammering. Block mod makes me question myself and my stammering and that is another of the technique's strengths. If I cannot manage any of the above in a given situation then I go away and ask myself why. I now seek out answers rather than wallow in the pit of self-induced despair. Once I have analysed my behaviour I come out fighting again. This ability to be self-analytical rather than self-critical has been developed through the use of block mod.

I am now my own therapist and have choices about the way in which I stammer. I couldn't ask for more than that.

Daniel Hunter

Mechanical devices

Sometimes people ask us if there are any devices they can use, either to make them fluent or to assist them in their talking. We rarely suggest their use because of the reasons below, but on occasions they can be helpful. We will briefly outline the most well-known of these devices, together with our thoughts on each.

The Edinburgh masker

This was all the rage in the late 1970s and early 1980s. It is a portable device comprised of a control box, a microphone and two earpieces. When a person wears the masker, they cannot hear their own voice as 'white noise' (a noise which blots out other sound) is transmitted to their ears. It is rarely used today. As you will see, the disadvantages outweigh the advantages.

Advantages

- Many people find they are fluent or much more fluent under these conditions.
- It may be useful for some people on some occasions when fluency is perceived as essential.

Disadvantages

- It only works when it is worn.
- It can have the effect of making the wearer look strange or different.
- When wearing the masker, it is often difficult to hear other people talking and thus it can impair communication. It can also be dangerous, for example, for pedestrians who cannot hear traffic noise.
- It does not work for some people.
- It can be very hard to put up with the noise in your ears every time you speak.
- It is only a crutch – nothing fundamental about the stammer or how you feel about yourself changes.
- It may only work for a time as people also learn to ignore it.

The delayed auditory feedback (DAF) machine

There are large, bench models and smaller portable models of this machine. Both work in the same way. The former is used for therapy sessions, the latter can be used in any situation. The mechanism is similar to that of the masker, but with the DAF machine, the speaker hears their own voice played back through the earphones very slightly after they have spoken. The amount of delay can be varied for the individual and the stage of therapy. To regain fluency, those using this machine produce a way of speaking akin to slowed speech (see under slowed speech earlier in this chapter) and this increases fluency. The main therapeutic use of DAF with people who stammer has therefore been as a way of helping them learn this technique. Some people have used it, however, in the same way as the masker.

Advantages

- Some people are fluent when wearing it.
- If slowed speech is the preferred technique, it can be helpful in teaching it.

Disadvantages

- Slowed speech is taught less often currently and, anyway, most people can learn it without using a DAF machine.
- Other disadvantages are as for the Edinburgh masker.

Metronome

The metronome is a device more usually associated with musicians, who use it to ensure they keep time when they are practising. Nowadays, these are electronic and send out an audible bleep at required intervals. In therapy, they were used to teach a way of speaking called *syllable timed* or *syllabic speech*, a very rhythmical way of speaking in which each syllable (or part) of the word is said with equal stress. It is rarely taught now.

Advantages

- It can demonstrate to those with very severe stammers that they can be fluent under certain conditions.

Disadvantages

- The speech produced sounds very strange – it has been described as being robot-like.

As you can probably guess, we do not encourage our clients to make use of electronic devices. We prefer them to learn techniques which give them real control over their talking, independent of any machinery.

Summary

Here we have been concerned with practical ways of changing your stammering behaviour. You may wish to experiment with some of these. If you wish to do so in any depth, we suggest that you consult a speech and language therapist. They can help you choose those techniques that are most suitable for you as an individual and help you to assess any groundwork which may need to be carried out before you embark on using them.

7

How can I best put myself across?
A guide to good communication skills

We have talked a lot so far about stammering, what it is and how to control it more effectively. However, communication is about much more than fluency, and more than talking, too. In this chapter, we want to look at three very important aspects of communication and at how improving these can increase your potential as a communicator. These are non-verbal communication, listening and assertiveness. These skills are relevant to all of us – people who stammer and people who don't. For some people who stammer, they may be particularly pertinent, for the reasons listed below. As you read them, ask yourself which, if any, apply to you personally.

- Because people who stammer often avoid talking, especially in certain situations, they can lack the experience necessary to build up a repertoire of communication skills. Some non-verbal skills, such as establishing eye contact or stating one's side of the argument – can get lost as the person panics about whether or not they will be able to say a particular word or worries over what the listener's reaction to their stammer will be.
- Fear of stammering often leads to people waiting for others to start conversations, relying on them to make or maintain relationships, make decisions, book outings and so on, rather than taking the initiative themselves.
- Many people find that stammering makes them feel different (often inferior) and this affects their ability to put themselves across in any other way. Their behaviour reflects the way they think about themselves. Thus, they may end up agreeing rather than disagreeing, holding themselves in a way which suggests a lack of confidence and so on.
- Much of the focus of the conversation can be taken up with thinking about fluency, the listener tending to be consigned to second place.

Non-verbal communication

Under this heading we include a variety of behaviours. We cover not only aspects of the way people look and act but also 'vocal' behaviours which complement the words they use, such as loudness and tunefulness. If you can

89

improve these aspects of your communication, you will find that the stammer takes on less significance as you are more able to see it as just one part of the total 'communication picture'.

Why is non-verbal behaviour important?

Non-verbal behaviour is used in a variety of ways. Here are just some of the more obvious ones.

- It is used instead of words – a glance or a shrug, for example, may be all that is needed to get a message across.
- It reinforces a message. The tone of voice we use, the intensity or otherwise of our eye contact, for example, can add important weight to the message we are trying to convey.
- It makes what we say more specific or complements the words. We might, for example, indicate size or shape using gesture. We may imitate someone to show exactly what they are like.
- It can also contradict the message the words are giving. A favourite example we often quote is of a politician (who shall be nameless!) we saw being asked a sensitive question on the television. The 'correct' answer was obviously 'yes', but the way he shook his head as he spoke the word showed that it was not what he actually believed!
- In a conversation, non-verbal clues are used to indicate whose turn it is to talk. We often lower our pitch and volume as we come to the end of what we are saying, thereby indicating to others that it is then their turn to speak.

Let's now take some examples of specific types of non-verbal behaviours. As we do so, think about your own use of them and consider how you could use our ideas to increase your skills in this area. As we said earlier, these skills are relevant to us all, whether we are fluent or stammer. However, here we aim to relate them to stammering.

Eye contact

Do you, like many people who stammer, find yourself avoiding eye contact, especially when you are stammering? If so, ask yourself why this is. Is it because you are embarrassed or ashamed of your stammer, you fear the other person's reaction, feel inferior to them or have just got into the habit of looking away when you talk to someone?

Next, ask yourself how other people might interpret poor eye contact. There are a number of possibilities. They may, for example, think that the person they are talking to is disinterested in them, bored, uncaring, unfriendly, shy, dishonest. This is probably far from how you actually feel, but your behaviour can suggest otherwise. Increasing your eye contact can help you to come across more accurately as the person you really are.

Another important factor to consider with regard to eye contact is that if you do not look at the person you are talking to, you are likely to miss some of the subtle messages they may be conveying to you, through their own non-verbal communication. If you do pick up on these messages, you are more likely to act appropriately. If, for example, the person looks bored, you need to change the topic or even end the conversation. If, however, they are smiling, you may wish to continue to entertain them!

The importance of eye contact becomes obvious if we notice the number of expressions which refer to it. A few which come to mind are 'he looked right through me', 'if looks could kill', 'he gave her the evil eye', 'he made eyes at her', 'she had stars in her eyes', 'they saw eye to eye'.

If you want to improve your eye contact, it may be easier to start by monitoring it when you are a listener. Do you have any difficulties in this respect? If so, perhaps this reflects the way you think about and value yourself with regard to others. Because you stammer, your self-esteem may be generally low. Try to value yourself more and realize that your stammer does not make you any worse (or indeed any better) a person than anyone else. If you do find that your eye contact is poor as a listener, start by trying to increase it in easier, more relaxed situations first. It may be, however, that your eye contact is only reduced when you are speaking, in which case you only need to work on it in this context.

Points to consider

- Good eye contact is not the same as staring.
- Increased eye contact tends to indicate increased dominance over someone or increased intimacy towards them.
- Decreased eye contact can suggest fear, lack of trustworthiness, shyness or thoughtfulness.
- The most effective sort of eye contact involves looking and then looking away for a brief moment.
- It is estimated that if you are to establish a good rapport with someone, your eyes should meet theirs for about 60 to 70 per cent of the time (Pease, 1984).
- The appropriate amount of eye contact varies according to the situation. In an interview across a desk with a bank manager, a lot of eye contact will be appropriate, whereas there will probably be little between strangers on a bus.
- One of our clients puts it this way, 'stammering merely tells people that you are dysfluent – eye contact says something about who you are'.

How to improve your eye contact

Become a good observer. Watch people having conversations and see how eye contact is used effectively and ineffectively and what this indicates.

- Monitor your eye contact in a number of conversations. Try to increase it little by little, starting with easier situations and gradually working up to more difficult ones.
- Set yourself tasks to help you to concentrate on the other person. For example, try to find out the colour, length and style of their hair, the size of their ears, the shape of their nose, the colour of their eyes and so on. In this way you are looking at the general facial area as opposed to staring into their eyes.
- Practise looking at yourself in a mirror as if your reflection is the person you are talking to.

Facial expressions

Facial expressions indicate how we feel. Some of the experts in this area say that these come second to the actual words in giving information to others, so they are obviously very important. Ask yourself about your own use of them. Do you have a limited range or use of expressions? If so, it may be because you are concentrating hard on trying to speak fluently or else because you find it hard to really relax in conversations and show what you are feeling.

Two main sorts of problems can occur with regard to facial expression. The first is that the face is blank or expressionless and so the listener finds it hard to judge what the person is feeling. The second occurs when the expression is different from what is actually felt. (One of us still remembers while at school being told that a teacher she liked had died. Her reaction was not to cry or even look upset but to smile from ear to ear, a reaction brought about by embarrassment and social ineptitude.)

Points to remember

- Several parts of the face are involved in facial expression. Brows can be raised or lowered, eyes widened or narrowed, nostrils flared or relaxed and lip position varied.
- Reflecting or mirroring someone's facial expression is a good way of showing you are listening to them.
- Increasing the scope and use of facial expression can help take the listener's focus away from the stammer and show that you are truly involved in what you are saying or are listening attentively.

How to improve your facial expressions

- Observe the range and variety of expressions that people use, the contexts in which they are used and what these different expressions mean.

- Try watching the television or a video with the sound turned down to see if you can work out from people's facial expressions what their moods are. Then, turn the sound up or replay the tape with the sound up to see if you were right.
- In a conversation, monitor your facial expressions when you respond. See if they indicated what you intended. If possible, ask others to give you feedback on this.
- Really concentrate on the content of what you and your listener are saying. When you take the emphasis off fluency and put it onto communication as a whole, you are more likely to respond with more appropriate expressions on your face. Your listener will feel better about you, too.

Gestures

Gestures are the movements we make as we communicate. They can involve various parts of the body – head, shoulders, arms and so on. Sometimes they are even used instead of speech. For example, a shrug of the shoulders may indicate that you are unconcerned or don't know something. They can also be used to accompany speech, either to stress a point (for example, when a fist is banged on a table to show anger) or to supplement a point (as when the hands are used to indicate size). Research has shown that gestures have five times the impact of verbal behaviours and if the two kinds of behaviours give different messages, it is the gesture which is most likely to be believed. Hence there is a lot of sense in working on the use of this kind of non-verbal behaviour.

Points to consider

- Sometimes people who stammer overuse gestures as a substitute for speech. Does this apply to you? Excessive gestures, fidgeting or fiddling, can be annoying to the listener and detract from what you are saying. They may also give the impression that you are feeling nervous.
- Other people underuse gestures as they feel anxious about communication as a whole and their gestures represent a form of distraction or avoidance. Are you more like this?
- However many or few gestures you use, you should feel that they help your communication as a whole. If they feel false, they will probably look false, too.

How to improve your use of gestures

- Become aware of how you use gestures – too many, too few or about right.
- Become aware of how others use gestures and of how you would like to be.

- Experiment with increasing or decreasing your use of gestures according to what you discover. If you notice you use too many, see what happens if you try for short periods to keep as still as possible. Find out which of your gestures aid your communication and which detract from it. Perhaps ask someone close to you to help in your observation. If you use too few, experiment with trying out some of the gestures you have seen others employ. Do not overdo this or you will feel and appear unnatural. Only use those gestures which aid you in communicating your feelings.

Posture

Posture is the term used to refer to the way we sit or stand. This can give an indication of how we are feeling. For example, we may slouch if we are tired or stand stiffly if we are feeling ill at ease. It can also be used as a way of demonstrating status. We can, for example, 'tower above' someone in power terms as well as height. If our posture is inappropriate, we can give out the wrong signals to the listener. For example, slouching may give the impression of sloppiness.

Points to consider

- The way you sit or stand can affect how confidently you come across, how others perceive you and, hence, also how you feel. If you stand or sit in a relaxed way with an open posture (arms and legs uncrossed), you are more likely to feel and be seen as confident than if you are rigid with a closed posture (arms and legs crossed or held tightly against your body).
- If you are leaning towards the other person, you are more likely to be deemed interested in them and in what they are talking about than if you are holding yourself back from them.

How to improve your posture

- Try to get a picture of yourself as others see you. Become aware of habitual postures that you adopt. Ask how they may be interpreted.
- Notice people around you who appear confident. What postures do they use which suggest this? If they said the same things but adopted different postures, would they come across in the same way?
- Be aware of how you can 'manipulate' your environment to your own advantage. For example, if someone who makes you feel unsure of yourself comes to talk to you and stands while you are sitting, equalize the situation by either suggesting they sit down or standing up yourself.

Vocal behaviours

Along with the words you use, there are other aspects of your talking which have an impact on how you come across. If you stammer, it is understandable that fluency is the aspect you may be most aware of and, of course, it is relevant. However, it is only one factor and should not be given sole importance. You can improve your communication by looking at your use of these other parts of speech and seeing if there is anything which needs altering. We will just say a little about each of them.

Volume

The loudness or quietness of your voice will affect your listener's view of you and the way they respond to you. Think of your own use of volume. Do you:

- vary the volume according to the situation (to take an extreme example, do you speak quietly in a concert hall and loudly in a crowded pub?)
- tend to use the same middle range in all situations, regardless of the subject matter, the person you are talking to and the situation you are in?
- speak loudly too often, in which case you may come across as domineering, bombastic or a loud mouth?
- speak quietly too often, in which case you may be seen as shy, self-effacing, unsure, in which case your listener can find it a strain to listen to you?

Points to consider

- Certain emotions tend to be associated with particular sorts of volume. Sadness and resignation are, for example, usually expressed at a low volume, whereas dominance and extroversion are allied to loudness.
- For those people who stammer and have a problem with volume, most speak too quietly. They may do so because they are concerned about stammering and use low volume as a way of trying to hide it. This can make listeners view them as nervous and unsure. It can also lead to demands for them to repeat what they have said and thus put extra stress on the speaker.
- Speaking at an appropriate volume can make you appear more confident and increase the listener's belief that you mean what you are saying.
- Increasing volume does not imply an increase in stammering.
- Occasionally we have met people who stammer who speak too loudly. It could be that they do so in order to appear more sure of themselves but have not monitored their volume closely enough and so have gone over the top.

How to improve your use of volume

- Monitor your volume in a variety of situations to see how appropriate it is. Ask others to tell you if you speak inappropriately loudly or softly.

- Notice if people often ask you to repeat what you have said. Sometimes people assume that this is happening because the stammer has made them difficult to understand, but more frequently it is because what is said is said at a low volume.
- Try to regulate your volume according to the person you are talking to, the situation you are in and the message you are trying to get across. It is no more appropriate to talk intimately to an ill person in a hospital ward in a loud voice than it is to give an order to a barman in a noisy bar in a whisper!
- Be aware that you are more likely to be seen as credible, interesting and sure of yourself if your volume matches the communication environment.

Tone, pitch, intonation and stress

Together these provide the 'tune' or the 'colour' in your speech. They give emphasis and interest to what you are saying. If you speak in a flat tone, at a constant pitch, with little rise and fall in your voice and no emphasis on particular words, not only will you sound boring, but your true meaning will not come across as effectively.

Points to consider

- We use different pitch and intonation patterns to convey different meanings. For example, we show we are handing over a conversational turn to someone by lowering our pitch and we indicate we are asking a question by a rising inflection. The use of such patterns can also be quite subtle. For example, we can say the same thing twice, but, using these patterns, either show that it is to be taken seriously or that it is a joke or a sarcastic remark.
- Vocal quality can have positive and negative implications. A thin voice is often associated with whining whereas a richer tone often indicates maturity or self-confidence.

How to improve vocal elements

- Thinking closely about the message you are trying to convey can help you use appropriate elements.
- An interesting exercise is to count to 20 and at the same time try to express different emotions. For example, count in a way which shows joy, anger, pleasure, annoyance and so on. Transfer what you have learned into real conversations.
- Another exercise is to say the same sentence so that it means something different each time. An example could be 'There are only 25 shopping days to Christmas' said as a statement, with amazement, panic, calmly, as

a question and stressing particular words (such as 'only', 'Christmas', 'are'), thus altering the meaning.

If you are interested in finding out more about this area, see the books listed in the Furthing reading section.

Listening

So far, we have looked mainly at your behaviours when you are speaking. Now, we want to move on to another very important part of communication – listening.

We have heard people who stammer say that because they spend more time than they might wish being silent, they are therefore good listeners. This may be the case for some, but we are aware that there are others whose listening skills are not good. This is, of course, just as true of people who do not stammer, for a variety of reasons. The following are just a few of them:

- the immediate environment is noisy or unpleasant (for example, smoke-filled) which makes concentration difficult;
- they are preoccupied, there are other things on their mind;
- they are not interested in the subject or the person;
- their previous experience – views, judgements, values, stereotypical thinking – gets in the way;
- they are selective in their listening – they only listen to things they are interested in, immediately understand and so on;
- they are short of time.

For those who stammer, there can be some additional reasons for listening being difficult.

Ask yourself if any of the following apply to you:

- you are so absorbed in planning what you are going to say next that you do not focus enough on the listener;
- you do not look at the person and so do not take in the non-verbal parts of their speech;
- you lose concentration as your turn approaches;
- you do not ask questions which show your interest because you are unsure if you will be fluent.

Communication is a two-way process. Thus, if you do not listen to the other person, it can become more like two monologues occurring in tandem. If this is an area you wish to work on, it is important to be aware that listening involves not only attending closely to what the other person is saying and doing, but also demonstrating that this is what you are doing in the following ways.

First, by your verbal responses:

- using words which reinforce what the person is saying – 'yes', 'mm', 'I see' and so on – which can be thought of as minimal prompts or cues which tell the person 'I'm hearing you, please continue';
- giving the person time to say what they have to without interrupting them or trying to take over the conversation;
- using similar language to show we are 'in tune' – not trying to impress, talk down to, shock and so on;
- keeping the movement of the conversation coherent – not moving on to a new topic out of the blue, but developing either the content or emotion expressed by the other person;
- referring back to things the person has mentioned or done earlier, such as 'You said it was Spain you went to on holiday last year' or 'You looked surprised when I mentioned X';
- reflecting back, as a question, words or phrases the person uses, such as 'he was worried?', 'she had eczema?';
- asking appropriate questions;
- summarizing what the person has said before you leave the conversational topic;
- accepting what the person says – this does not mean you have to agree with what they say, but that you accept it as their view and are not judgemental.

Second, by your non-verbal responses:

- keeping appropriate eye contact but not staring;
- using facial expressions which reflect what the person has said
- sitting or standing in a relaxed way;
- nodding, shaking your head and so on to show your feelings without interrupting the person's flow;
- not using distracting behaviours, such as fiddling with a pen or a ring, fidgeting or looking at something else in the room;
- not being afraid to keep silent, rather than rushing to fill gaps in the conversation.

By keeping these factors in mind and perhaps by asking for feedback, you can quite quickly identify any areas of difficulty in your listening skills and try to incorporate any new behaviours.

Assertiveness

The final area we want to explore is one which we have heard many people who stammer (and many who do not!) say they have difficulty with. It is also one about which there is often some confusion, so we will start by finding out what the term 'assertiveness' actually means. We will then go on to look briefly at what the skills of assertiveness are and at how you can improve your performance in this area. Unfortunately it has to be 'briefly', because in the space available we can only touch the surface of this important area. We have therefore listed several useful books in the Further reading section to which you can refer if you wish to explore this area more.

What is assertiveness

Every book on assertiveness attempts to define the term in its own way. We do not propose to give yet another definition, but rather say simply that it involves the following areas:

- feeling good about yourself;
- feeling equal to others and acknowledging that others are equal to you;
- being able to put forward your opinions openly and honestly and listening to what others feel and think;
- taking responsibility for yourself and your actions.

Assertiveness does not imply getting your own way at all costs. Assertive people can admit that they are wrong, give way to others' better judgement and apologize when they need to. The outcome of assertiveness is that no one's rights are violated and no one feels oppressed.

Let's compare assertiveness with two other ways of being, namely non-assertive and aggressive. Non-assertive people do not stand up for themselves. They often do not express themselves, believing they have little to offer. If they say their piece, it is frequently apologetically and hesitantly. They see the rights and views of others as being more important than their own. Aggressive people, on the other hand, stand up for themselves so much that they violate the right of others to do the same. They dominate and often domineer.

The differences between these three sorts of behaviours become clearer with an example. Person A asks person B a favour. To comply with the request would be possible but create all sorts of difficulties for B. Here are B's three possible responses.

The aggressive person: 'How can I possibly do such a thing? It's out of the question. You'll have to find some other idiot to do it.'

The non-assertive person: 'It's a little bit difficult, but of course I can do it for you.'

The assertive person: 'I'd help if I could, but on this occasion I have to say no as it would really muck up what I've planned for myself today.'

How to be assertive

- 'Own' what you say by using the word 'I', but not in a way which compromises others' rights.
- Seek out, listen to and properly consider the views of others before making up your mind.
- State what you have to say clearly and succinctly.
- Be prepared to disagree, but also to change your mind if the other person's opinions are more convincing.
- Do not confuse fact with opinion.
- Use body language which matches the words you are speaking.
- Be prepared to make and admit to making mistakes.
- Avoid using words like 'should', 'ought' and 'must', but, rather, use 'could, 'want, and 'can'.
- Say 'no' without feeling guilty. Do not say 'yes' when you really mean 'no'. Be honest about your reasons.
- Ask people for favours, but accept that they may be unable or unwilling to oblige.
- Accept and give criticism in a constructive way.
- Do not tell others how to behave.
- Neither boast, nor put yourself down.
- Use a clear voice and speak at a steady rate.
- Avoid the use of threats, blame or excessive sarcasm.

A comment

As a person who has stammered since the age of 8 (I am now 34), I experienced many years of being stared at, laughed at and receiving that 'blank' look from the person I was trying desperately to speak to.

These reactions, occurring on a regular basis, have had an effect. They have made me feel less confident in my abilities, whether concerned with speech or not. They have also made me feel the need for approval from others – 'Did I do that well?', 'Do they think I'm slow?' For many years I totally avoided the telephone – it's amazing what technology you can do without! In time, I began to view myself as a stammerer *first* and my own person *second*.

Assertiveness can be defined as the art of clear, honest and direct communication. This may appear difficult at first for someone who stammers but it can be achieved. The first thing is to believe that you are a person who happens to have a stammer. Some people have eye squints, some have oddly shaped features – all sorts of differences which make us human. However, speech is a bit different because it may not be obvious at first and people you are talking to can't always hide their reactions when the stammer occurs.

For me, the best way of overcoming this has been to explain to people on first meeting that I have a stammer – then it's out in the open. 'I'd just like to explain I've got a stammer but don't let it worry you. If I get stuck on a word please wait – I'll get there!' As a result, I can concentrate on *what* I'm saying, rather than *how* I'm saying it. Sometimes I stammer less because I'm not as anxious about doing it.

This approach usually has another positive effect – it makes listeners less embarrassed. It also gives them the opportunity to talk to you about stammering; it helps others understand. Assertiveness gives you the freedom to be who you are, not who other people think you are – their misjudgements may be based on the fact that you stammer. That is unfair and needs to be addressed. For me, assertiveness has been one way of doing this.

Maria Neary

Summary

In this chapter, we have looked at three important areas which can greatly enhance the effectiveness of your communication. We are aware that we have only really skimmed the surface of these. There are several ways of finding out more. You can read the books we recommend in the Bibliography, you can contact local education centres which put on courses on subjects such as confidence building, assertiveness and effective communication, and many speech and language therapists, especially those specializing in dysfluency, are able to offer advice and training in these areas.

8

How can others help me?

In this chapter we will look at a number of the treatment options available to those of you who are considering seeking help. Where we can, we will give details of the professional background and approaches used in the different therapies. There are some, however, on which we have been unable to gather any specific information and these we include for the sake of completeness.

Speech and language therapy

A speech and language therapist is someone who has undergone a period of undergraduate study, usually of three or four years' duration. The degree course itself is validated by the 'host' university and the Royal College of Speech and Language Therapists, and as such has to contain certain components, including many hours of teaching on stammering and other fluency problems and clinical practice outside the university.

On completion of the degree, a therapist then registers with the Royal College of Speech and Language Therapists and is qualified to practise in any setting. This registration also carries with it insurance for the therapist, access to a professional journal, contact with other therapists and a commitment from the therapist to further develop their skills and level of competencies. A speech and language therapist may work in a number of different settings. They are usually based in a community clinic or hospital, but may also carry out consultancy work in schools and other educational establishments.

There are a number of speech and language therapists in the United Kingdom who specialize in fluency problems. These therapists have usually undergone further training and may have learnt additional skills in areas such as psychology and counselling. They will almost certainly be members of a special interest group which meets on a regular basis to discuss issues in stammering and keeps up to date with current trends in treatment and theory. If you are seeking a speech and language therapist to discuss and treat your stammer, it is definitely worth checking whether or not they are a specialist and, if not, where one could be located.

Since the inception of their profession, speech and language therapists have been associated with the treatment of people who stammer. Much has changed since those early days – we no longer advocate painful surgery to the tongue, singing what you wish to say or speaking like a dalek to a rhythmical beat. Specialist therapists offer a wide range of therapy procedures which are tailored to suit an individual's needs. For example, specific techniques related to breathing or relaxation may be recommended if the person is found to have a poor breathing pattern and excess tension when speaking. On the other hand, if someone is finding stammering difficult to cope with, a combination of counselling, desensitization and cognitive therapy might be agreed. The therapist will take a detailed history of the problem, assess the person's difficulties and then discuss with the client what options are available. In many cases, group therapy programmes are a popular approach. This is not seen as a cheaper alternative to individual therapy, but has actually been found to be a more effective treatment in the long run for many people. There are many types of group programmes. Generally they can be divided into two broad categories – those in which all the group members follow the same series of steps in sequence at roughly the same time and those in which people meet as a group but work on separate tasks, progressing at their own rate. There are advantages and disadvantages to both approaches, but those seeking a group therapy programme should consider which one is best suited to their difficulties and learning style and discuss this with the therapist.

It is worth pointing out that many specialist speech and language therapists have established close links with self-help groups in their area and with the British Stammering Association. Indeed, a number of therapists act in an advisory capacity for the Association. This contact works to the benefit of both parties as it enables professional opinion to be coupled with the views of the users of the service. We will discuss the British Stammering Association in more detail later in this chapter.

If you wish to be seen by a speech and language therapist, then the procedure is quite simple. An open referral system is in operation, which means that you can contact a therapist yourself and ask for an appointment. Alternatively, you can request a referral from your own doctor or, in the case of children, from a health visitor, teacher or nursery nurse.

A national directory of therapists can be found at the offices of the Royal College of Speech and Language Therapists in London (see Useful addresses at the end of the book), and the British Stammering Association also has detailed information about specialist services in certain areas of the country. Specific information about therapy and therapists in your locality is available from your local health services, hospital or community trust headquarters, or the speech and language therapy manager, also entitled head of service in some places.

Psychological approaches

Psychological approaches to stammering have been used to treat people who stammer for at least as long ago as the time of the famous Freud. In his day, stammering was viewed in a variety of ways, including as an 'oral fixation', an 'anal fixation' and a 'compulsive neurosis'! It was generally believed that there was some kind of 'inner conflict' responsible for stammering. It was thought that if this could be treated, then the 'symptom' of stammering would be cured. However, this approach did not appear to be very successful and people who stammered tended to be viewed as highly resistant.

Things have changed a lot since then. Nowadays, the psychological components of stammering are generally seen not as the *cause* of the stammer but as a *result* of it. People are viewed as individuals who have reacted to stammering in a variety of different ways and, thus, may need differing degrees of psychological help as a part of their therapy. How much they need will depend on how the stammer has affected them and on events in their lives.

Counselling and psychotherapy

These are descriptive terms for 'talking therapies'. There is much controversy as to the differences between the two, but, generally, counselling is shorter, deals with the 'here and now' and goes less deeply into a person's past than does psychotherapy.

The theoretical approaches used are many and varied. The scope of this book does not allow us to explore this in any great depth, but we can perhaps give you just a taste of those used most commonly in the treatment of stammering.

Personal construct therapy (PCT)

This approach began to be used with people who stammer after 1972 when the psychologist Fay Fransella wrote a book entitled *Personal Change and Reconstruction* (1972) describing how she had applied it with a number of her clients.

Personal construct therapists see stammering as something a person does because they understand stammering more than fluency; they make sense of the world through their 'stammering eyes'. The approach is a very optimistic one, however, and there is a belief that people can learn to see stammering differently and make more personal sense of fluency.

By means of particular techniques, such as 'self-characterizations' and 'repertory grids', therapists enable people to change their 'construing' of their stammering. This may involve, for example, learning to view themselves as people who stammer rather than seeing the stammer as being the most important factor or discovering that others do not see the stammer as negatively as they do.

Cognitive therapy

This is a relatively new form of therapy and one which is gaining in popularity and availability.

Cognitive therapists look at how people's thoughts influence their actions and feelings. The aim is to identify negative thoughts, help clients test out their validity and replace these with more useful thoughts. Cognitive therapists believe that thoughts are only thoughts, not reality.

Methods used in this form of therapy include the keeping of diaries, rating the strengths of someone's beliefs in a variety of situations and carrying out experiments in the clinic and between sessions to try out new behaviours.

Solution-focused brief therapy

This kind of therapy looks at solutions rather than problems. In fact, some brief therapists say they do not need to know what a client's problem is in order to help them solve it. Therapists work with clients to identify those times when the problem is not happening and discover what it is they are doing which is preventing it from occurring. The client is invited to picture very closely how their life would be without the problem and then explore how this alternative way of being can become a reality.

These are only three of many approaches currently in use. If you are interested in pursuing this area you can take one of several routes:

- More and more speech and language therapists, especially those who are specialists in dysfluency, are trained in counselling, and they will discuss your needs in line with their own training and approaches.
- Your GP may be able to refer you to a counsellor or psychotherapist working in the NHS, or some GP practices employ their own counsellors, as do some of the larger employers.
- The British Association for Counselling (BAC) provides lists of private counsellors in specific geographical areas, giving details of their qualifications and the types of therapy they offer (see Useful addresses at the end of the book and write to them for a list, enclosing a SAE).

Many private counsellors offer a sliding scale of charges according to clients' earnings. In many cases you will be asked to sign a written contract which outlines areas such as confidentiality, number of appointments, cancellations and so on. All reputable counsellors receive supervision of their practice to ensure that they are working in clients' best interests.

Most counselling or psychotherapy sessions last for around an hour. The number of sessions you will need to attend will vary according to the approach used and what it is you are hoping to achieve.

If you opt for private therapy, we suggest you go through a bona fide organization, such as the BAC. Anyone can set up as a counsellor, so it is important that you satisfy yourself that the person you see is qualified and practising ethically (see comments on this elsewhere in this chapter).

The BAC publishes a very useful booklet entitled *Counselling and Psychotherapy: Is it for me?* This describes counselling in straightforward language and looks at the differences between counselling and psychotherapy and where they are available. It outlines a little of what you might expect when you go for therapy, including what might happen in a first interview. Finally, it gives an idea of questions you might ask to ensure a therapist has the appropriate qualifications and experience and works in an ethical way.

Self-help

There are burgeoning numbers of self-help groups for adults across the United Kingdom. These have largely grown up since the 1980s, with the help of the British Stammering Association, and now operate in most areas of the country. In a survey carried out in 1987, Bryan Hunt (a member of the British Stammering Association) found out several interesting facts about the groups running at that time:

- The age range of members was between 25 and 40.
- Groups were generally small, with usually four to six members attending as a rule.
- Meetings were usually held weekly, but some were fortnightly or monthly to suit the membership.
- Most groups started when therapy groups had come to the end of a programme of therapy and members wanted to continue to meet or, occasionally, they formed when people left one area and were looking for support in the area they had moved to.
- Activities varied from group to group – speech-related activities were common, such as practice of fluency techniques learnt in therapy, role-playing job interviews, reading aloud, quiz games, giving talks and so on.

In the past we, as speech and language therapists, have tended to use local self-help groups as 'holding bays', as it were, for clients awaiting therapy and then, at a later stage, for clients who have completed a course of therapy.

These days we would recommend that clients join a self-help group and continue membership while they are engaged in speech therapy. (We have luckily had the goodwill of the Leeds group, which has changed its meeting night to accommodate members attending the speech therapy group.)

We know that self-help group membership is not for everyone – some people just do not like joining groups. To paraphrase something Groucho Marx once said, 'I would not want to be a member of any group that had me as a member!' Some feel that joining a group of this type separates people from the society they desperately wish to be a part of. However, we believe that, for others, the self-help group can be a lifeline. In reviewing his survey, Hunt concluded that self-help groups offered a number of short- to medium-term benefits – social contact with others who stammered, new insights into the nature of stammering and the development of helping strategies for members, in the absence of competition with more fluent speakers. Our experience with the group in Leeds would lead us to agree with Hunt's conclusions. We would particularly note the help it offers in terms of reduced isolation and add that the self-help group provides a safe haven in which to practise any techniques or tasks and receive constructive, informed feedback. It can often be a lot of fun, too!

Medication

We often wish we had a little pink pill to give to those coming to our clinics in search of a quick route to fluency. Unfortunately, we do not, nor indeed do other people. However, a number of drugs have been and are prescribed by some doctors to alleviate some of the symptoms. Most of them can be categorized as stimulants, sedatives or tranquillizers, and they act by changing the biochemical composition of different parts of the nervous system. (Paradoxically, the same classes of drugs can also be employed to *induce* stammering in adults!)

The use of medication is not advocated as a *cure* (that is, to eliminate stammering), but it has been used on its own and in conjunction with other therapies to *control* some symptoms, such as tension, negative emotions and anxiety. In general, the research on the effectiveness of drugs used in treatment is inconclusive. For some people, there is no effect, but for others there can be changes in the severity but no reduction in the number of occurrences of stammering. These findings should be interpreted cautiously, as many of the studies were carried out on small numbers and not always with adequate controls. Remember, too, that the effects only last while the person is taking the medication, and these effects must be weighed up against the long-term side-effects which many of these drugs carry with them.

Alternative therapies

There are increasing numbers of people, keen to rid themselves of stammering, who have become dissatisfied with more conventional methods of treatment and are looking for alternative approaches. We shall now review several of these alternatives and, where possible, assess what they might have to offer the adult who stammers.

Hypnosis and hypnotherapy

The hypnotic state has been defined as one which involves both a psychological and a neurophysiological element. Thus, under hypnosis, changes are said to occur in feelings and bodily sensations. There is considerable debate as to whether or not a hypnotic or trance-like state actually exists. It is a very subjective experience and, therefore, it is very hard to define what is happening when someone is hypnotized. However, what can be agreed is that the phenomenon is brought about by the suggestions of another person – the hypnotherapist in the case of therapy or the client themselves in self-hypnosis.

Hypnosis, then, is a state of changed awareness associated with deep relaxation. While in this altered condition, various procedures and techniques can be used (this is the *therapy* part of hypno*therapy*). These include the following:

- Deepening – increasing the level of relaxation.
- Ego strengthening – a type of confidence-boosting procedure in which suggestions are made to the person to the effect that previously difficult situations will be easier to cope with.
- Anchoring – holding on to good, positive feelings.
- Regression – a person is encouraged to remember or re-enact experiences from their past which are thought to be significant, perhaps even a cause of their current difficulty.
- Post-hypnotic suggestion – the person is taught to regain the hypnotic state on presentation of a 'cue', like a touch of the therapist's hand or a verbal command.
- Auto-hypnosis – teaching someone how to bring about a hypnotic state themselves, while remaining in control and alert at all times.

Most therapists agree that a rigorous assessment procedure should take place to decide whether or not hypnosis or hypnotherapy is a suitable procedure for the person wanting it. It is clear that this treatment is not appropriate for everyone. One writer lists a number of conditions which would be contra-indicators. These include mental illness (such as schizophrenia) and brain tumours (Waxman, 1989). Other factors which may be significant are said to be the strength of the person's commitment to therapy, the level of their motivation to change and how well the therapist prepares them for hypnosis.

There is certainly some evidence of hypnosis and hypnotherapy being used with adults who stammer. Indeed, there are some speech and language therapists who are trained in its use. The research on hypnotherapy with adults who stammer is limited, but most professionals would agree that hypnosis alone will not be enough to make a long-term difference to a person's speech. Nevertheless, it may be a useful tool to promote calm and relaxation. This said, hypnotherapy can be effective when it is used in conjunction with some speech therapy techniques. Some research has shown that it can be effective when treating anxiety which occurs in speaking situations, to eliminate or control extra movements of the body or face which sometimes accompany stammering and when teaching block controlling techniques. It is, however, a tool and, to our knowledge, has as yet never 'cured' stammering.

Most hynotherapists are independent practitioners, although there are one or two who are employed by health authorities and/or GPs. Charges are usually per session and several sessions may be recommended to treat stammering. Contact the BSA in the first instance for more information about this therapy as treatment for a stammer and how to go about finding a suitable therapist in your area (see Useful addresses at the end of the book).

Acupuncture

Acupuncture is founded in traditional Chinese medicine. This type of medicine is based on the belief that illnesses come about as a result of imbalances in the body and a combination of factors such as diet, stress, time of the year or seasons. The aim of acupuncture is to treat the individual by looking at these various factors. Different acupuncturists adopt different approaches. Some will take a symptomatic approach, treating the symptoms that a person reports, while others take a more holistic view and treat body, mind and spirit. Disorders are thought to result from problems in life energy pathways, with different problems arising from specific pathway deficiencies. The pathway is cleared by the insertion of an acupuncture needle and electrical energy flows are stimulated. With regard to stammering, the fire element is thought to be involved, particularly the heart energy pathway. Thus, acupuncture needles would be inserted along the course of this pathway.

Someone attending an acupuncture clinic for the first time will undergo a diagnostic session, lasting up to one and a half hours. During this time a full history will be taken, including details of medical history, but also childhood experiences, how the body is functioning and so on, and the 12 Chinese pulses will be read. In subsequent therapy sessions, following a brief review of how the person has been feeling since the previous session, the acupuncture needles will be inserted at the appropriate points. Of the 360-plus classical acupuncture points, those below the elbow and below the knee (approximately 70 to 80) are commonly used. In any one session three, five or seven points will be used. Points are usually 'moxaed', that is heat is applied, either directly onto the surface of the skin or via the needle. (In certain circumstances – for example when a person has high blood pressure – moxaed needles are not recommended.) The needles may be applied and then removed very quickly or can be left in situ for approximately 20 minutes. The sensations that follow treatment have been described as a dull ache. With some points the feelings are a little more painful, but the discomfort is momentary. Treatment is usually in the form of one session per week. Progress is reviewed after a number of attendances and clients are expected to see some change after seven or eight treatments. Thereafter, people may return to their acupuncturist for 'top up' sessions at the change of the seasons, when different points (energy pathways) may be relevant to their condition.

In treating long-standing stammering in adults, most acupuncturists we have talked to feel that they have something to offer, but treatment may well involve attending for sessions over a prolonged period of time. They admit that the stammer, in these cases, may not be 'cured', in the sense that it would disappear altogether, but it would be less frequent and/or less severe and the person would feel more able to deal with it. It is worth noting that several acupuncturists report that those they have treated have experienced additional unforeseen benefits from their treatment, such as better levels of energy, improved sleeping patterns and more satisfactory interactions with other people.

The Alexander technique

This approach is based on the work and writings of F. M. Alexander. Alexander developed a voice problem while he was working as a professional reciter of dramatic pieces. His doctor recommended resting his voice before his performances, but this did nothing to alleviate the problem. His difficulties became so acute that, even after following the doctor's orders, his voice deteriorated to a hoarse whisper during an important recitation. At this point Alexander began to look at ways to cure himself.

He started by comparing his behaviour during performance conditions with that in normal speaking situations, comparing what he was doing when the problem was there with when it was absent. His initial detailed observations revealed differences in the position of his head and larynx and, later, he noted differences in his spinal position and stance. Alexander taught himself to acquire greater control over these aspects of his behaviour and, as a result, found that his voice problem was cured.

In writing of the application of this technique to other problems, he documents the case of someone with a stammer (one of a number he says he treated). He describes stammering as 'the misdirection of the use of the psycho-physical mechanisms', and treats it in the same way as he does other difficulties, by improving the alignment of the spine and how the limbs are held in relation to the spine.

Homoeopathy

Our knowledge regarding the homoeopathic treatments for stammering is limited. However, for the purposes of this book, we have made contact with a number of centres in our locality. It is clear that they are rarely asked to treat stammering in isolation and, indeed, would not do so as it goes against the philosophy of this approach. Homoeopaths believe in treating the *whole* person and would, therefore, carry out a full assessment of all symptoms, which may or may not include stammering speech.

We suggest that if you are interested in this form of treatment, you contact a local homoeopathy clinic and discuss your symptoms with the therapist.

As an aside, we were recently made aware of the theory and practice of Bach flower remedies (a recommended text on this subject is *Bach Flower Therapy* by Mechthild Scheffer). A number of substances were recommended as being useful for people who stammer, including cherry plum, to manage the fear of speaking, vervain, to promote relaxation, and rock water, to lessen self-criticism.

It should be noted that neither of us has any experience with either homoeopathy or Bach flower remedies. We therefore merely present these to you as options which are available, but we cannot comment on their effectiveness.

How do I choose a therapy that is right for me?

As you can see, a variety of treatments is currently on offer, many with accompanying claims of greatly improved speech and lifestyle, and it is difficult for the average person to separate out genuine from spurious help. In our book *Helping Children Cope with Stammering* (also published by Sheldon Press, in 1996) we discussed some of the concerns we had about a number of individuals and agencies offering therapy for those who stammer. For this reason, we included several issues to consider when choosing a treatment regime and we repeat these for you below as we believe these are as relevant to adults who stammer as they are to parents seeking therapy for their children.

- Is the therapist or organization registered in some way and are they registered with a professional body that has a code of ethics to which each member must adhere?
- Does the therapist hold qualifications which are accredited by a professional body or institution?
- Is the therapist or organization offering more than their own first-hand experiences?
- If the therapist or organization intends to see you and offer you some form of therapy, are they (and you) covered by an insurance policy?
- Are you clear about what the therapist or organization is able to do for you? Is there any evidence available that they can do what they claim? For example, can you talk to anyone who has undergone the same or similar treatment?
- Does the person or organization have up-to-date knowledge about stammering in adults, or have they been offering the same approach for a number of years without modification?
- Is some form of follow-up programme offered after treatment?
- Does the British Stammering Association have any knowledge or experience of the programme or on what information the therapist or organization is offering? (Does it check out?)

9

Coping with difficult reactions
and tricky situations

In this chapter we want to look at what you can do when people react in a way which you find unhelpful or when you are in a situation where you find it hard to speak. Our aim is to help you approach and not avoid these problems and then to find strategies which work for you. This is not an easy task because everyone is different. For a start, the things that bother one person may seem a doddle to another and vice versa. In addition, what may be the best way of dealing with a difficulty for one person may not work for another. However, the good news is that, having met hundreds of people who stammer over the 20 years we have worked with the client group in Leeds, we have a good idea of the main areas of difficulty and some of the ways that seem to help. We suggest you focus on those areas that are relevant to you. In terms of solutions to the problems, we propose to offer some choices. You can then experiment and find those that suit you best.

Difficult reactions

Emotions

Here we will list some of the negative emotions some fluent people can have towards people who stammer. However, in doing so we do not want to suggest that the majority of people you speak to will see you in a negative light because you stammer. Some will, but many will view your speech as just one aspect of your whole personality. In addition, people are generally genuinely interested in stammering. As we have mentioned elsewhere in this book, we find people we meet are very keen to discuss stammering when they discover what we do for a living.

Here are some of the more negative emotions we commonly hear about from our clients.

Embarrassment

You may feel that some people appear embarrassed when they are talking to you. While we know this may occasionally be the case, we suggest you ask yourself why you think it is so. Sometimes in response to this question our clients say it is shown in the way the person looks or in their averted gaze when they stammer. However, we notice that some of the clients who offer these explanations always avert their own eyes when they stammer, so we ask them whether they are really able to judge this accurately. We also suggest that they consider whether their listener is embarrassed because of the stammer or because of the embarrassment of the person who stammers. That sounds rather complicated so we'll explain it a bit more. Imagine you are talking to someone and you want to come across well. Your stammer is quite severe and you feel embarrassed, wondering what they will be thinking about you. In your embarrassment, you shuffle about, fidget with your hands and look away every time you start to stammer. The listener picks up your embarrassment and starts to feel embarrassed, too. In other words, it is your *embarrassment* and not your *stammer* which has caused your listener's embarrassment. In either case, what can you do? Here are some suggestions:

- Keep eye contact when you stammer. This way you will look more confident and in control while keeping the channels of communication open.
- Mention your stammer to put the other person more at ease and to show you are not embarrassed about it yourself. This prevents the 'game' which is often played – a person stammers, acts as if they haven't, in such a way that it tells their listener that they are not to show that they have noticed the stammer. The listener tries to oblige, but ends up not knowing how to react. However, when the person who stammers acknowledges their stammer, either directly (for example, 'My stammer is quite severe today') or indirectly ('That was a difficult word to say'), the listener is given permission to notice it and, ironically, is less likely either to notice or be embarrassed.
- Accept that some people are embarrassed by stammering, as people can be by anyone who is different from them. Do not take responsibility for their embarrassment. Instead, try to show them that they do not need to behave in this way by not allowing it to affect you. Continue to say the things you want to.
- With some listeners, you may feel able to talk about their embarrassment openly. You could say something along the lines of, 'You seem embarrassed when I speak to you. You don't need to be. My stammer doesn't embarrass me.' The appropriateness of these comments, of course, depends on the situation and the other people involved.
- We have occasionally known of cases where the close relatives of someone who stammers are embarrassed when the person stammers in front of certain people, for example strangers or close friends. They often anticipate a reaction in these people which may not happen. We have

heard of relatives who, for example, nudge someone in an attempt to stop them talking in such situations. This can be very upsetting. The advice we would give here is to try to bring this out into the open as soon as possible, discuss it, explain the effect it has on you and ask for the person's co-operation in reacting differently. Don't be intimidated – see it as a challenge!

Pity

It is a normal human reaction to feel sorry for someone who has a problem of some sort. Ask yourself who you feel sorry for. Is it your friend whose partner has died, the man down the road who has cancer or is in a wheelchair, or your child who hasn't got a best friend? Often this is the way we express the caring side of our natures. When we are on the receiving end, however, we frequently see it differently. We feel put down, undervalued or misunderstood. We say, 'I don't want them to feel sorry for me', but usually we do want them to care about us. It's a difficult position for the person to get just right! What then should you do if you believe someone is feeling sorry for you?

- Sometimes it can be helpful to consider what is behind the emotion. Is it genuine care or is it a feeling of superiority or contempt? If it is the former, ask yourself if you really need to be disturbed by the reaction.
- If the pity is less than caring, try to use your assertiveness skills to show that you have no reason to be thought of in this way. You may well stammer, but you have rights like everyone else. You can still say the things you want to, even if it takes you a little longer.
- Remember that if you back down by stopping talking or using avoidance tactics in the face of this reaction, then you have, in effect, let the other person 'win'.

Treating you as if you were stupid

We have clients who say others react to them as if they are 'not all there' or at least not as intelligent as they really are. We have wondered if this belief is carried over from schooldays, when the child behaved in such a way so as not to show their ability to the full because they did not want to stammer in front of everyone. You may remember doing these things yourself – not answering questions in class, pretending you didn't know the answer to a simple question, saying you didn't do your English homework in case the teacher asked you to read out your story and so on. Perhaps you are expecting people to think like this because you allowed them to in the past and assume that this is a universal reaction. Now ask yourself if you still do things which hide your true ability, rather than risk letting others hear your stammer. Think about those things for a minute and see if this is true for you. If so, why should people react as if you were brighter than you show them you are? How can you prevent such a reaction occurring?

- Ask yourself if you are judging the person fairly or whether you are making assumptions because of your previous experience.
- Say the things you want to – do not avoid doing so for fear of stammering. The listener will not know this is what you are doing and could just think you don't know the answer or got it wrong.
- Tell the listener you stammer and will need more time, but that you do have something to say on the subject. In this way you can disprove their belief in your lack of ability.

Anger

Occasionally people report that others have become annoyed or even angry with them when they have stammered. This reaction may be grounded in frustration or in the belief that the person is stammering on purpose and could actually stop it if they wanted to. On other occasions it is not the stammer they are really reacting to but something else. Most of us know how easy it is to take our frustrations out on the wrong person when it is not possible to do so on the one who really deserves it – like when the boss does something unfair to you and your partner suddenly finds that they can't do a thing right all that evening! It is a fact of life that some people are not as tolerant or as patient as others and they may find your stammer frustrating to listen to, especially when it is particularly severe or they are in a hurry and can't spare the time to listen. Here are some things you can do which will help:

- If the person is someone you know well, explain that stammering is not something you do deliberately – you are not a masochist! However, the more you try to control it by 'pushing through' words or using avoidance tactics, the worse it will get. Ask them to help you and tell them the things they can do. If they can take a positive role in helping you, they may find it easier.
- Try to be forgiving when the anger comes as a result of a 'final straw' on a bad day.
- Try not to take the anger personally. It is caused by frustration at your stammer and you are not your stammer. We guess you feel angry with it yourself sometimes, so why shouldn't others?
- If it is a stranger who gets angry, be assertive. We have heard of people being told to 'spit it out' or 'get on with it, I haven't got all day'. It's

amazing how some prolonged eye contact and a particular type of facial expression can undermine such people! A remark can have a similar effect. For example, one along the lines of 'I wish I could, but I have a stammer' or ' I would if I could but, having a stammer, I don't have the way with words that you seem to.'

Condescension

One of the reactions clients have told us they find most infuriating is when people treat them in a patronizing way, as if they are 'poor little things' who cannot manage themselves and need to be helped out. Perhaps if this is something you feel, once again you need to ask yourself if this is actually what the person is feeling. Often people are really trying to help but are unsure how to. Maybe they have never met anyone who stammers before and don't know how to be helpful. They want to make it easy for you to talk to them, but just try too hard. And some people are like this with everyone – stammer or no stammer! If you experience this kind of reaction, here are some things to consider:

- Ask yourself whether or not the reaction is a well-meaning one.
- Consider whether or not this person would react to you in this way if you did not stammer.
- Show by your behaviour that this kind of reaction is not warranted – use good eye contact, a confident posture and say the things you want to.
- It may be appropriate to mention the stammer, to show them you are in charge and to give them an alternative way of reacting. For example, you could say, 'I have a stammer and you can help me best if you just wait for me to finish what I am saying.'
- Don't let their reaction get you down. You may not be able to alter the person, especially if this is a way they commonly behave. However, you do not need to take responsibility for their behaviour.

Behaviours

As well as particular emotions people may display with those who stammer, there are also some behaviours that can be difficult to deal with. Here, we shall look at some examples of those we are told about most often, again offering suggestions as to how to deal with them which we hope you will find helpful.

Finishing your words

We frequently hear how irritating many people who stammer find it when others finish what they are saying for them. While there are some who do not object to this kind of intervention, most seem to. This is for a number of reasons. For a start, the person knows what they want to say; it just takes them a little longer to do so than others. The listener may also get it wrong and then it will be necessary to correct and clarify the point, which can take the conversation right away from where it was going originally. The listener is also taking control away from the speaker. As a result, there can be pressure on the person who stammers either to say the next difficult words they come across as quickly as possible, struggle to force them out or avoid saying them altogether.

There are several ways of dealing with this sort of behaviour:

- Through your non-verbal behaviour (by maintaining good eye contact, relaxed posture), you can show the person that you are endeavouring to say the word and are keeping calm in your attempt. In that way, the listener is less likely to feel the need to step in to rescue you.
- You can tell the person that you would prefer them to let you finish the word yourself. You do not need to be aggressive – indeed, you may thank them for trying to help, but offer them an alternative way of doing so. For example, you could say, 'I know you are trying to help, but, actually, I would prefer it if you just waited until I have said the word, rather than say it for me.'
- Ignore the word filled in by the listener and just carry on as if they have said nothing. They will soon get the message!

Interruptions

There are some people who will interrupt others at any opportunity. This is regardless of whether the person stammers or not. There are others who will interrupt those who stammer, perhaps through embarrassment, because they do not know how to react appropriately, or to try to prevent them from being hurt by an adverse reaction. We know this can be very frustrating.

The ways of dealing with this sort of reaction are similar to those given for dealing with someone who finishes your words, with a few adjustments:

- Use your non-verbal behaviour to show the person that you intend to carry on claiming your turn until you have finished what you have to say. Look the person straight in the eye and, perhaps, touch them on the arm, as if to restrain them from speaking.
- Tell the person you have not yet finished what you are saying.
- Act as if the interruption has not occurred and just keep talking.
- Tell the person that it helps your speaking most if they can listen while you are talking and interruptions make it harder for you.

Offering suggestions

It is not uncommon for others, especially those close to you, to give you their 'wisdom' as to how you might speak more fluently. High on the list of *good ideas* are 'slow down', 'take a deep breath' and 'calm down'. If only it were that easy! Sometimes the advice is to say another word – something you are hopefully working to *stop* doing.

Once again, these suggestions are usually made with the best of motives and people do genuinely want to help. Occasionally, however, the reactions are born out of lack of patience, poor listening, frustration, a bad day at work and so on.

Here are some suggestions for dealing with unhelpful advice.

- Tell the person that the advice is inappropriate. For example, 'It really doesn't help me to take a deep breath – in fact it's more likely to make my speech worse.' You might feel it helpful to preface this with, 'I know you are only trying to help, but . . .' Another way of saying the same thing is to say, 'I just wish it was as simple as that. I've been trying it for years but there's been no success so far!' You could refer to your speech and language therapy or even to this book. For example, 'It's funny you should tell me to try and say another word because that's just what my therapist says I must stop doing!'
- Give the person a specific role in helping you. For example, you might say, 'Telling me to calm down usually only makes me more tense. However, I'd find it really helpful if you could point out when you notice me clenching my fists/biting my lip/stamping my foot. I'm trying hard to work on that, but find it difficult to notice every time I do it and could do with some help.'
- Tell yourself the person is trying to help in the only way they know. You know it doesn't help and can therefore choose to ignore it.

Laughing at you

Laughter at stammering usually occurs because of embarrassment or ignorance. It can be very difficult to tolerate, though, and it is easy and natural to let it upset you. Often it brings back memories of those worst of times at school when stammering made you the butt of people's jokes or unkindness. What should you do about this kind of reaction when you are an adult? Here are some ideas:

- It is important to remind yourself that, although the same emotions may be triggered, this is not the same situation as when you were a child. Doing this can prevent you from reacting in the same way as you did then, perhaps by withdrawing, becoming upset or retaliating, possibly aggressively.

- Being assertive can be a very effective put-down, especially if you feel the laughter was maliciously intended. Saying things such as, 'Actually, I have a stammer and it is difficult for me if you laugh when I speak' can put the cleverest of clever Dicks in their place!
- Behaving as if the person has not reacted in this way can stop the person continuing to act in the same way. Maintaining eye contact, smiling, keeping calm and even voluntarily stammering can show the person that their reaction has no effect on you and you are not going to be put off your stride.

Not respecting you as a person

Under the heading Embarrassment at the beginning of this chapter you will recall that we mentioned how people might look away when they talk to you. They may ignore you in other ways, too. For example, by addressing their remarks to someone you are with rather than to you (this is sometimes referred to as a 'Does he take sugar?' reaction) or keeping conversations short.

You can deal with this by taking the following actions:

- Keeping eye contact yourself.
- Answering directly the remark addressed to the other person.
- Being up front about your stammer, so the person feels less awkward.
- Not being intimidated but saying all you have to, regardless of the reaction you receive.
- Asking them to direct any remarks about you to you personally.

Not giving you the opportunity to do things or overprotecting you

We have known people who prevent the person who stammers from saying or doing the things they want to. This is often done with the best of intentions, but sometimes from less positive motives. A negative motivation is usually linked with embarrassment, as we discussed at the beginning of this chapter. A positive motivation for such a response often stems from wanting to protect the person who stammers from being hurt and so this problem usually arises in relationships with your nearest and dearest.

The best way to deal with this is to be open and honest and tell the person who is doing this something like, 'I have been running away from my stammer for years and trying to pretend I am fluent. This tactic has meant I have not really said the things I want to and have avoided many situations where I think I might stammer. I need to change that now, but I can't if you continue to try to overprotect me or do and say things for me. I know I have probably encouraged you to do those things in the past, but I'm trying to take control now. If I need help I'll tell you, but otherwise I want to have a go at things myself.'

Tricky situations

Here we will look at situations which our clients tell us can be particularly difficult to deal with because of their stammer. Again, we will offer some ideas that might help you to deal with these situations more effectively.

Speaking to strangers

Are you one of those people who finds speaking to strangers especially troublesome? If so, this is probably because you fear the sort of reaction you might receive if and when you start to stammer. Does it often feel as if you spend the conversation waiting to stammer and, indeed, when you do, is it almost a relief that your 'guilty secret' is out in the open?

There are a number of ways in which you can ease the stress of such an encounter:

- Do not try to hide the stammer. The more you hide it, the more tense you are likely to become and the less natural and enjoyable your conversation will be. Accept the fact that you stammer, and think about what you are saying and what your listener is saying to you. Show the person you are not concerned or embarrassed by your stammer and it is less likely that they will be.
- Admit that you stammer. Tell the person. This can often give them 'permission' to notice and, ironically, they are then likely to notice it less.
- Use voluntary stammering to show the person that you stammer, but also that you can be in control. You should do this early on in the conversation to reduce your anxiety level.
- Concentrate on your communication skills as a whole instead of just thinking about your stammer.
- Be assertive and take control of the situation. Don't let the other person make all the running. Don't be passive and wait for them to ask you questions. Take the initiative, asking questions, steering the conversation in ways you want it to go, rather than panicking about how you will respond.

Speaking to people in authority

Does talking to the boss, or other authority figures, fill you with horror? If so, why is this? Is it because you feel that they will judge you negatively? Do you think you will stammer more severely or not be able to put your point across in this situation? For whatever reason, many people who stammer find this sort of conversation difficult (as indeed do many people who do not stammer).

Here are some ideas for coping more effectively with such situations:

- Take your time. Do not give in to any urge to speak as quickly as possible to get the conversation over with.
- Concentrate on what you are saying, not on how fluently you are saying it. Aim to come over as an interesting person with good ideas rather than as a fluent but somewhat boring speaker.
- Use good communication skills to help you express yourself as confidently as possible. Pay particular attention to maintaining good eye contact so that you appear trustworthy and self-assured.
- Think positively. Tell yourself that just because this person holds a higher rank than you it does not mean that they are any better a person.

Asking for tickets and speaking in a queue

These two speaking events are similar so we will look at the most helpful ways of dealing with them together.

The act of asking for a ticket is often complicated by several other factors which can make talking more difficult, such as talking through a grille and having to say something specific. In addition, there is frequently a queue. Sometimes in both these activities there is also time pressure and there may be increased background noise, too.

Here are some ideas you may find it helpful to use to tackle such situations successfully:

- Try to focus on the person you are talking to. In doing so, aim to cut out the other people around you from your thoughts and even from your field of vision. Just think about talking to the one person as if no one else exists. Concentrate on that person, what they look like, the mood they seem to be in, their voice – anything that helps take the emphasis away from what you have to say and/or your fear of stammering.
- Speak slowly and clearly. In this way you are most likely to be heard straight away and so will not have to repeat yourself. Do not respond to time pressure by speeding up – instead, 'make haste slowly' as one of our clients said!
- Try to be prepared and reasonably sure of what you want to say. However, do not be overprepared (for example, do not rehearse the exact words to say) or inflexible. If so, you may find it hard to adapt if things go differently from how you have planned.

- Talk positively to yourself. For example, in your head, say, 'I am in control, I am relaxed and calm.' Talk yourself into success, not out of it. Remember, the person you are talking to is going to be more concerned about taking your money than about whether or not you stammer!
- Use good eye contact as then you show the person you are beginning to engage them in conversation, even if you do not actually start to speak as soon as you would hope.
- Remember your rights. You are not stammering deliberately (unless, of course, you are stammering voluntarily!) and it is your right to expect the other person to wait for you to say what you want to. If the listener is impatient, unkind or whatever, it is their problem, not yours. Remind yourself of this.
- The object of the exercise is to get your ticket. If you end up with what you want, the encounter has been a success, regardless of how you have spoken.
- In queues, use the waiting time to concentrate on relaxing, perhaps going through various muscle groups to check that they are not becoming tense and to consciously relax them if they are becoming tight (see Appendix II for a relaxation exercise to try).

Talking in a group

This activity worries many people who stammer, and many who don't. Often it is a situation someone who stammers avoids as far as possible, and so their difficulty is worsened by lack of experience. Noise often compounds the problems they face.

There are several ways of dealing with talking in groups, including the following:

- You may find it helpful to talk mainly to one person, perhaps someone you can see or hear easily, someone you feel at ease with or with whom you have discussed your stammer.
- It can be easier to address your remarks to no one in particular but to use good general eye contact to show the audience that you are talking to all of them.
- It is often very helpful to tell people about your speech difficulty, either as individuals or as a group. If this is too difficult to contemplate just now, consider asking someone else to ensure that everyone knows you have a stammer. In this way you don't have to worry about whether or not you will surprise people by stammering as they will know in advance.
- Do not put more demands on your speaking than you feel able to deal with. You do not always need to be the life and soul of the party. Say as much as

you feel comfortable with. Sometimes this will be more than at other times. Try to increase the amount you say as you become more confident. Count your successes, not your failures.

Ordering in a restaurant or at a bar

Some people who stammer avoid this sort of activity completely. Others only order things they know they can say, which of course limits them considerably. Yet others rely on those they are with to do the ordering and may thus feel inadequate or foolish. In addition, friends may see them as mean if they do not offer to buy a round and so on.

So, what can you do if you want to change?

- If you recognize these scenarios, ask yourself why you are more concerned about stammering than about these other things. Is it really preferable to eat a salad when you yearn for chilli or to let friends judge you falsely when you hold back from offering to pay? What would actually happen if you went ahead and did stammer? Would people really judge you so harshly? Does the waiter or barman really care if you stammer? Try it out once in a 'safe' situation, with your nearest and dearest. It is likely that you will be far more fluent than you anticipate, but even if you do stammer you are likely to find that people's reactions are far less negative than you imagined they would be.
- Experiment in small steps (remember the hierarchy idea in Chapter 4, under the heading Taking small steps). Start off, for example, by asking for one course or drink in a bar, café or restaurant which is uncrowded and friendly. Repeat this process until you can do it without feeling anxious. Your aim should not be to say it fluently but to say the thing you want. Only once you can ask with low anxiety should you try a slightly more difficult task.
- Enlist the help of others. Explain your difficulty to the people you are with. Tell them how hard it is for you, but that you are working to change.

Saying important words

Inevitably on occasions you will find yourself panicking because you have to say particular words which you are unable to avoid. Names, addresses, telephone numbers, dates of birth all come into this category. Having said that, we have known people who have still avoided some of these things and given false answers, including a different name!

Assuming you want to give the correct information, what should you do?

- Don't panic! This will only make things worse, but of course this is easier to say than to do.

- Don't expect to be fluent. Make it your aim to get the information across in whatever way you can.
- Pause and establish eye contact before you start to speak.
- Keep your speech unhurried. Use any speech techniques you find helpful to achieve this.
- Use voluntary stammering on a non-feared word leading up to the one you fear.
- Admit that you stammer and perhaps tell the listener that you find it particularly difficult to say the word you are attempting. Ask them to wait and be patient.
- See under the heading A comment, following the discussion of easy onset, Chapter 6.

Talking on the phone

This is one of the situations many people who stammer find most difficult. The big difference between speaking to someone face to face and speaking on the phone is that on the phone you cannot see the person. Thus you have only your speech to rely on and your non-verbal communication cannot be used to help you. Sometimes the listener does not hear you stammer but is aware of silences, which they may not understand. At other times, they may hear the stammer but not know how to react. Perhaps they hear the stammer and react in a way which is unhelpful or even rude.

Over the years, while working with people who stammer, we have discussed with them practical ideas for making it easier to use the phone. We include those ideas here, but you need to experiment and find the ones that are appropriate for you.

Becoming desensitized Some people find themselves panicking at the mere sound of the phone or at the thought of picking up the phone. A useful aid here is a process known as *flooding*. In practice this means immersing yourself in a task until the anxiety you experience subsides. You may, for example:

- record the sound of the phone ringing and play it back to yourself over and over until it no longer affects you;
- practise just walking up to the phone until this can be done without anxiety, then the next step could be to pick up the phone without saying anything before moving on to picking it up and saying 'hello' or your name;
- let the phone ring a little longer than usual before you pick it up.

Repeat these activities until they no longer cause you concern.

Answering the phone

- Take your time. It is easy when you feel panicked to rush at picking up the phone and blurt your greeting out as quickly as possible in order to try and get the words out fluently. Very often, though, this has the opposite effect and you become tense and stammer severely. Instead, try to get into the habit of answering in a slower, more relaxed way. When you hear the phone, let it ring a few times before answering. Walk up to it slowly and pick it up in a leisurely way. Make sure you do not hold the phone tightly and thus create tension in your body. Watching yourself in the mirror as you phone can help you monitor tension.
- Pause momentarily before you start to speak. This enables you to compose yourself and calm down. Say your greeting slowly.
- Don't force yourself to answer using a particular set of words. Sometimes, for example, people feel they must say their telephone number when this is really difficult for them and 'hello' would be much easier. You can still experiment with different ways of answering, but don't put pressure on yourself only to answer in one way and in a way that is difficult for you. Telephoning can be hard enough – you don't need to make it even harder.
- Encourage your partner, child or colleague not to answer the phone but to let you do so. In this way you will increase your experience of speaking on the phone.

Making a phone call Now we will look at several phases of making a call – preparing to make a call, making the call, ending the call and coping with difficult listeners.

Here's how you can go about preparing to make a call:

- Think of a good time to make the call – when you have just had a row is not a good time, for example, nor is when someone else is waiting to make a call! Try to do it when you need to – putting it off only serves to build up the pressure. Don't make the call when you are in a hurry; ensure you have enough time.
- If you can, make the call without an audience. If this is not possible, then think only about the person you are talking to. Blot the audience out, turning away from them if you can.
- Picture the person you are talking to. Try to imagine you are talking face-to-face with them and don't stop yourself from using non-verbal communication (smiles, gestures and so on). Picturing them as being a sympathetic listener can be helpful. If you are phoning someone who

makes you feel on edge, it can be helpful to picture them sitting in their underwear, not in smart clothes!

- Ensure you are sitting in a relaxed and comfortable way, holding the phone gently.
- Have an idea of what you want to say, but don't plan it too closely. You cannot predict what the person on the other end will say and if you overplan you can be thrown if things don't go as you expect them to. If you have quite a lot you need to say, you might find it helpful to make some notes beforehand as a guide and so that you do not omit anything important. It may be useful to have a paper and pencil handy if you need to remember anything or want to jot down something you might wish to respond to later in the call.
- If you have avoided the phone but want to start using it, build up a hierarchy (see section in Chapter 4 on small steps) of calls. Start by making the easiest until you only feel low anxiety when you do it. Then try the next easiest call in the same way and gradually work up the hierarchy. Repeat the easier calls even when you are working on the more difficult ones as this will help increase your sense of confidence and mastery. When you reach the more difficult calls, you may wish to find some *Freefone* numbers to ring if you don't want to work up an enormous phone bill! Our clients have found that phoning for car insurance quotes is a good way of practising those things they find especially hard, such as speaking to strangers, giving specific information (their name, address and so on) and answering rapid-fire questions.
- Make more calls when your fluency is at its best – enjoy them!

How can you make it easier on yourself to make a call?

- Start off by speaking a little more slowly, making the first sound very gently with a light contact (see under the heading Speed of speech and pausing, Chapter 6).
- Monitor your level of tension throughout the call, keeping as relaxed as possible. Check, for example, that you don't hold the phone tightly, scrunch your shoulders up and so on.
- Press the numbers slowly, taking your time. Some people find it helpful to say the numbers aloud slowly as they press them.
- Use voluntary stammering if this is something you are familiar with (see under that section in Chapter 6). By allowing yourself to stammer early on in the conversation, you can stop worrying about when your listener will find out your 'guilty secret'. It can also make you feel more in control.

- Consider telling listeners that you stammer and let them know how they can help you. However, do not apologize for your stammer. Instead, you might say something like, 'I have a stammer and it would help me if you could give me time to say what I have to.' Our clients tell us that they generally receive very positive responses to such requests. Listeners usually feel better when they understand the reason for the pauses in the conversation and have an idea of how best to react.
- Try to keep your speech slow and clear. In this way you are more likely to stay in control.
- Don't spend the call trying not to stammer. If you just let the stammers out they are less likely to become really tense.
- Think about the message you are trying to convey, rather than dwell on your dysfluency. Do not judge the success of the call on whether or not you were fluent, but rather on whether or not you said what you wanted to and achieved your purpose.
- Don't make assumptions. If your listener is abrupt, unresponsive, unhelpful, it is probably nothing to do with your stammer and may be nothing to do with you – perhaps they have had a bad day, you have got them at a bad time or they are eating their tea or watching the television as they are speaking to you!

Now let's look at how you can tackle ending the call:

- You may find it helpful to have a 'winding down' phrase to prepare the other person for the fact that you are going to ring off soon. Phrases like, 'It's been nice talking to you', 'When will I see you next?' and 'I must let you go now' can be useful.
- You can thank the person if they have responded in the way you wanted them to. They are then more likely to behave appropriately with you another time or with someone else who stammers on the phone.
- Vary the words you use to close the conversation. Don't make the task more difficult by forcing yourself to say particular words.

You are bound to come across difficult listeners. Different people find different responses problematical. Here we list just a few with some possible solutions, many of them thought up by our clients during workshops we have run on using the phone.

For a person who says little or gives little feedback:

- check they are still there and have not been cut off (if they are there, this may help them realize what they are doing);

- mention to them that you wonder what they are thinking as they are so quiet;
- be open about your stammering and how you want them to respond – they may be doing nothing for fear of doing the wrong thing;
- don't take responsibility for their response, just for your own;
- ask a direct, open question which demands a response from them.

For a poor listener:

- check out their understanding of what you have said;
- if they talk a lot, either wait until they have finished and say your piece or use a phrase like, 'I need to tell you something' to establish your turn;
- tell them about your stammer and how you need time to speak;
- if you are interrupted, say, 'Can I just finish?'

For someone who is abrupt:

- check out if there is a reason – they may be in the middle of something or in a rush, for example;
- ask if you can ring them back at a more convenient time;
- keep calm and don't take responsibility;
- let off steam after the call is over!

Summary

In this chapter we have looked at people and situations which can make talking especially difficult. We hope you have been able to identify the difficulties you experience personally and found some techniques you think could be interesting to experiment with. There are no right answers – you just have to find those that help you best as an individual. Try to ensure, however, that any methods you use entail being open and bring your stammer to the surface, rather than hide it.

10

Maintaining positive change

It is a well-known fact that changing your speech is relatively easy, but that the harder part is keeping that change going over time. Then there is the really, really hard part – when you have to use your new skills in those situations where you usually expect to stammer and/or where you need to be open about your stammering. Because we know that this is likely to be difficult, we need to consider what you need to do before you actually reach that point.

Keeping change going

First of all, we would like to review those things that help to maintain change. We will summarize these points here, but you may want to reread the fuller discussion of them towards the end of Chapter 4.

- Continue to experiment with change. Try out new things from time to time, just for the fun of it.
- 'Loosen' your way of approaching new behaviours and situations. That is, try to think about them and act in ways which enable you to have choices. For example, approach situations by replacing 'I can't do X. I have never done X before and I am not going to start now' with 'Well, I'll try X just this once. I might like it, I might not, but I will not know until I have given it a go.'
- Work on new things by taking small steps.
- Talk to yourself in a positive way and give yourself little rewards.
- Be open with other people and involve them in helping you to maintain the positive changes you have managed to achieve when this seems appropriate.

Maintenance skills

As we mentioned earlier in the book, each of the clients who attends our therapy programme leaves with their own, tailor-made 'toolbox'. This is a collection of strategies, ideas and techniques accumulated during therapy, which they know will help them to maintain the skills they have developed. Now we shall look at some of the tools mentioned in the literature on the subject of maintaining change and others which have proved most popular with our clients.

Problem-solving skills

When you have difficulty with a particular speaking situation or person, then it is useful to approach the problem as you might do any problem in life. There has been some helpful work carried out in this area in the past and we have devised a ten-point plan drawing on the results of this work.

Step 1: define the problem

At the beginning it is necessary for you to be clear about what the difficulty actually is. It is not enough simply to say, 'I have problems saying my name.' That is too big a statement and one that needs to be broken down until you have precise details in order for it to be usefully tackled. You should try to define when and where the difficulty occurs – the time of day, who else is involved, what your emotional state is at the time and so on. So, you might end up with a definition something like this: 'I have trouble saying my name first thing in the morning when I feel half asleep and have not worked out precisely what I want to say on the phone to someone important whom I have never met when others are listening to my conversation.'

Step 2: identify problem areas

Have a go at working out what is causing the difficulty. At this stage, you may or may not come up with any answers, but that is not actually the aim. What you are working at is developing a more critical, objective approach to your difficulty and trying hard to remove the emotion. Not an easy task we know! Taking our example from step 1, the problem areas could be drawn from this list:

- poor concentration;
- need to impress;
- lack of preparedness;
- lack of speech practice (this may be the first speech of the day);
- a specific word needs to be said;
- tiredness;
- fear of the phone;
- who, in particular, is listening to your call.

Step 3: analyse those times when there is no problem

At a guess, we would suspect that your stammer is not there all the time. For instance, there are probably times when the client in our example can say their name. In step 3 you need to spend some time thinking about those

131

occasions when the problem is absent. Consider what is happening at such times, what it is that makes the experience a better one with regard to stammering. Was anyone else involved, did you feel differently? If you are able to identify any important differences then perhaps these can be applied to improve the problem times.

Step 4: find possible solutions

This step involves brainstorming all the possible ways of solving the difficulty. It is important at this stage that you keep an open mind and include *all* options, good and bad. Don't worry about how you feel about each of the possibilities – that comes later. Again, using our, by now familiar, example, *their* list may look like this:

- get someone else to make the call;
- wait until I have woken up;
- get a good night's sleep;
- leave them to guess my name;
- write a letter;
- go somewhere else to make the call;
- tell them 'I can't say my name';
- write my name down and read it over the phone;
- use a different name each time;
- make some practice calls to people I know and can say my name to;
- use a fax machine;
- tell them I have a stammer and find saying my name a problem;
- change my job to one where I don't have to use the phone;
- e-mail them;
- pretend I have forgotten my name;
- do some talking before I make the phone call.

Step 5: test options

Now is your opportunity to test out the possible solutions to the problem. First, make a list of the solutions, starting with the most appealing and ending with the least attractive. Then, beginning with the first option, devise a little plan to test out its usefulness. The number of steps required will depend on your plan of action. For example:

- preferred option no.1:
  - make some practice calls to friends before I make the call:
  - explain the problem to Bob and Megan
  - check that they are willing to be involved, will take it seriously, can take a call before 9 am and will give me honest feedback

- agree a trial of five separate days
- write a reminder in my diary and put Post-it notes about it on my computer screen at work
- tell Isla that I'm going to do it (then I won't bottle out)
- do it five times!

Step 6: record key learning points

It is no use doing the testing without recording the results, so step 6 is all about writing down what you have learnt from each of your 'experiments'. Try to record your observations as soon after the test as possible and in as much detail as you can, then you are more likely to recall all the aspects.

Step 7: write an action plan

On the basis of your experiments, you should now be in a position to know what works to solve your problem. It may need some fine-tuning, but the rudimentary elements will be there.

You should now write a plan of action, indicating the details of what you are going to do and when you propose to implement the changes. For example:

> Starting on Monday I am going to get up ten minutes early each working day. I will talk to the radio in the car to get some talking done before I arrive at work. I am going to prepare what I have to say to my important caller before I ring them up. If I get stuck on my name, I'll tell them that I have a stammer and sometimes have difficulty with my name.

Step 8: make refinements

Plans do not always work on the first attempt and we have to continue to learn from our experiences. Step 8 is concerned with reviewing the plan after an appropriate time. When you do this you will need to consider which aspects have worked well and which ones need to be revised.

Step 9: rewrite the plan

Leading seamlessly from step 8, after revision comes rewriting. Thus, the issues which have been learned from a period of reflection are incorporated into a new improved plan of action, again with full details and an implementation date.

Step 10: learn from problem solving

The final step of this approach is to try and take an overview of problem solving as a whole. What did you learn from the way you tackled this particular difficulty? Did you rush any stage? Did you benefit especially from any one step? Were the plans you formulated detailed enough? Do you think you are developing a more analytical approach to problems – if not, how might you work on this area? To complete the exercise, make a note of things you have learnt and put it somewhere where you will find it the next time you have a problem to solve.

Managing the bad times

One of the fundamental aspects of any maintenance kit is having some tools to manage the bad times. Let us be realistic, there will be some bad times (or at least occasions which do not live up to our expectations!). We need to plan our strategies for these eventualities before they occur, so that we can weather the storm rather than catch cold in it!

Our clients are especially good at devising tools for this part of their kit and we have learnt much from them. Here is a selection of their ideas and one or two of our own.

'Jewel' card

Write down on a small piece of card a number of memories which you can look back on with pride and fondness. These may be events, experiences, achievements, something someone said to you, a smile from someone you cared about – anything at all, big or small. These are your 'jewels'. During the bad times or perhaps in situations where you need to lift your spirits, take out your jewels and spend a few moments going through them and enjoying recalling them. Let yourself feel the positive emotion that they produce before returning the card to your pocket or other safe place.

Reward yourself

If you receive a reward after a particular behaviour, you are more likely to perform the same behaviour again at a later date. This is quite a well-known piece of psychological theory which you could make use of in your toolbox. If you have tried something new or done something which has been quite difficult, give yourself a reward. Not only have you earned it, but it will mean you are more likely to try the same thing again later. The reward does not have to be a big one – something like a bar of chocolate or a long soak in a lovely warm bath are fine. It could be fun to contemplate the reward you might choose!

A 'toolbox' reminder

This is a bit like the jewel card only this time on the card you have a list of everything in your toolbox. When things are going badly it can be hard to remember what to do. Sometimes the negative emotions take over and it is difficult to see a way out. Carrying the toolbox reminder card around with you can help to get you back on the track again, and there might be a particular tool that you had forgotten about – you never know.

Give yourself permission to stammer

Sometimes, even when times are rough, we have the same high expectations of ourselves. We rarely adjust our anticipations to match the demands of the moment. So it is with stammering. If your speech is going through a bad patch, it may be because there are a lot of other things in your life generally which are difficult to manage. In these situations, it is hardly surprising that your speech is not so good, but do not go back to your old habits. Instead, show yourself some understanding. Think, 'Today is not as good as I know I can be, but that's OK, given the rest of the things I am coping with. I need to take extra care of myself and my speech and look at my toolbox to see what I should do.'

Give yourself permission to worry

It is OK to be concerned about situations as long as the worrying does not prevent you from functioning. During difficult phases, try limiting your worrying to a set time. For example, from 7 to 7.15 or on the train home. During this period allow yourself to worry like mad, just let it all happen. Then, at the end of the allotted time, you must stop worrying. Even if you have not finished, even if you have not had enough time to worry about X, the worrying must end at that moment and you must move on.

Positive self-thinking

You may have noticed that throughout this book we have not referred to people who stammer as 'stammerers'. This is a positive decision on our part and one which reflects our beliefs. A person who has a stammer is much more than the stammer – your speech is not the sum total of who you are. So, when your speech is not all you hope it might be, remember, there is a whole lot more to you than the way you speak.

Remember, too, that you have a number of strategies which you can use to control your speech. Your speech does not have to control you. Use your knowledge about stammering. People who stammer know a lot about stammering, both from their own personal experiences and often from the literature on the problem. When your speech is bad, think about what you know about stammering – how variable it can be, what tends to make speech good, what situations and events can cause it to take a nose dive and so on. Go over what you know in your mind's eye and try to see how the current dark days fit into this knowledgeable perspective.

Concentrate on the present

It is easy to worry, we know, but try to keep your anxieties in the here and now. Then they are easier to manage. You cannot affect the past but you may very well be able to do something about what is happening in the present. Avoid the 'What if . . . ?' thoughts and focus your energies on where they can best be used.

Balance the negative thoughts with the positives

Negative thoughts can be destructive, sometimes eating away at your self-confidence and your view of yourself. We recommend that you work on nurturing more positive and encouraging messages for yourself. Experiment with alternatives and see which ones feel best. Then, when a negative thought pops into your head, such as, 'I never come across well in this situation', take it out or shut it out by replacing it with one of your 'positives', such as, 'I know most people get nervous in this type of situation. Today I am going to try and say what I really want to and keep avoidance at a minimum. If I can achieve this, then I will feel I have succeeded and will give myself a little treat.'

Confront the fear

When an issue or event is bothering you and you are having difficulty putting it out of your thoughts, then face up to it. Ask yourself why it is of such concern. What is it about the situation that is such a problem? Try to imagine the worst thing that could happen to you and think about all the possible things you might do if your worst imaginings were realized. Often people find that the worst thing they can imagine is not so terrible and they actually have a number of tools in their toolkit that they can use to manage it.

Techniques and practice

One thing about life is that it rarely stays the same, so the chances are that your speech, and your ability to control it, will vary, too. You have to be prepared for these variations, and some of the ideas in this section will help you manage them.

Self-monitoring

One of the first things we suggested you did in this book was to get to know your stammer. You need to be thoroughly acquainted with it in order to recognize what goes wrong. This monitoring should be an ongoing process.

In order for you to be able to keep monitoring, you will need to vary how you do it. This helps to keep you on your toes and on the look-out for changes in the pattern of your speech. Here are some options for you to consider:

- Keep a fluency diary. Record your speech – the good and the bad – and think, especially, about why the good times went well.
- Use a dictaphone to record samples of your speech in certain situations. Remember to play the tape back and be constructive in your self-criticism. (Note that you should tell other people that you are recording if you intend to tape their speech in addition to your own.)
- Plan your self-monitoring at the beginning of the week. Choose a different situation or a different time each week to keep you on your toes. You may need to make a timetable or record the times in a diary to remind yourself to do it.

Practice

It is important to practice, of that there is no doubt. Practice ensures that new-found skills are kept honed for when they are required. There are some key factors to remember about any practice you do:

- You can practice a skill alone, but this will never be enough. The best sort of practice is that which takes place in a speaking situation with other people, where you have to work on the skill in conjunction with all the other communication skills you use – eye contact, facial expressions, listening to the other person and so on.
- Keep your self-monitoring objective – imagine you are listening to a total stranger.
- Base your practice on your self-monitoring. Identify what you need to work on and then plan your practice accordingly.
- Do not forget to work on good communication skills in general terms, including all those mentioned in Chapter 7. This will take the pressure off any need to be fluent.
- Be systematic in your practice, working from the easier to the harder levels, and record your progress.
- Short periods of practice spread across a day are better than one long session which happens infrequently.
- Look back over your therapy notes from time to time and/or read about stammering, especially the experiences of others who stammer.
- Talk to other people about your practice, enlisting their help if it is appropriate.
- Vary your practice so you don't get bored.
- Plan your practice sessions ahead of time.

- Build on your successes. Try out new speaking situations and keep taking risks.

Each person must decide for themselves how they incorporate practice into their routines. There is no one answer for everyone. Again, we will make a few suggestions and then you can experiment to find the one that suits you best.

- Set aside 20–30 minutes per day, divided into sessions across the day, such as 10 minutes first thing in the morning, 10 minutes over lunch and 10 minutes last thing at night.
- Crisis practice – that is, practice one or two critical skills before an important speaking event or when stammering is likely to occur.
- Tailor-made practice – that is, matching the practice to observations made in your fluency diary or other self-monitoring. For example, you may have noticed from your observation tapes that you were speaking in a hurried way. This will alert you to the need to practice speaking with a greater number of pauses and/or at a slower speed. Your tailor-made practice may then be telling your children a bedtime story at a slower speed and with more pausing as you do so.

Using triggers

We have both had personal experience of trying to remember to do something which is outside our normal routine – and having failed in the attempt! It is hard. Sometimes having a reminder, or 'trigger', in place is a good way of helping the memory along. Many of our clients have devised ingenious ways of cueing themselves in to the use of a technique – Post-it notes, messages in an (electronic) diary, drawings on the fridge, an elastic band around the wrist (for the duration of an important situation), putting their watch on their other wrist (again for the duration required) and setting the alarm on their digital watch. Choose one of these and see if it works, if not choose another or, even better, make up your own! Change the reminders from time to time or they will become habits and cease to remind you.

Personal care programme

It is important to see your speech as one part of the whole you. In which case, it is no use taking care of just one aspect of you and neglecting the rest. Any toolbox, if it is to be of any lasting use, should include good maintenance tools for the whole person. Think about:

- exercise;
- sleep;
- diet;
- relaxation.

We suggest that you do lots of exercises, particularly for your speech muscles – talk as much as you can, use every opportunity to speak, seek out new speaking situations and boldly go . . . !

Support systems

You need a good support system. The tools in your kit may require overhauling and servicing from time to time and you must know where to go to get this attention. People vary in the type of support they find useful – you may have one person who you can rely on to be there when you need them or, perhaps, you like a group of friends around you in times of trouble. You may find a self-help group for people who stammer or the British Stammering Association useful options. Speech and language therapists are usually willing, on request, to provide 'top-up' sessions and/or review how you are progressing. Whatever your preference, ensure that it is worked out before the need arises.

Some final thoughts

Finally, to conclude this chapter, we would like to quote from Breitenfeldt and Lorenz (1989), who summarize many of the key factors about maintenance (we have adapted some of what they say to meet the needs of this book, but the sense remains unaltered).

Life after therapy
One type of therapy may be over, but a new phase is beginning, a phase which will require a different commitment from you. We would urge you to consider a number of issues as you embark upon your 'life after therapy'.

Fear of stammering
Continue your openness about stammering – show your stammering and talk about your stammering with others. Confront your stammer when you are with family, friends, colleagues, strangers, people who you think do not know about your stammer, people on whom you wish to make a good impression and people you would like to show how fluently you can talk. There are different ways of facing the fear of stammering, for example:

- tell people that you stammer;
- discuss what stammering means for you with other people;
- make a comment about your speech when you are dysfluent and/or when you are using a controlling technique;
- use voluntary stammering;
- use feared words and sounds;
- work any substituted or avoided words back into sentences as soon as you realize that you have avoided them;
- cancel your biggest dysfluencies.

Controlling the fear

Remember that stammering is something you do, not something that just happens and over which you have no control:

- whenever you fear stammering in a particular situation, use voluntary stammering and advertise your stammering to others;
- whenever you go into a new situation, it is advisable to use voluntary stammering as soon as you can (if you do not use it early in the conversation, you may be tempted to try and be a non-stammerer), use voluntary stammering whenever you find yourself not wanting to stammer and, remember, a lot of stammering is what you do to avoid stammering;
- use voluntary stammering when you are having a fluent period – this will keep the fear of stammering at bay and help you when you feel you are skating on thin ice;
- use light contacts of your speech structures when you anticipate a dysfluency;
- when you are stammering, remember to move forward in your speech;
- try not to return to any old habits of managing stammering, such as forcing the sound out or pushing through the blocks.

Socializing

Continue to work on your social skills. Do not just do those things that come along by chance, but manufacture situations yourself. Get out and make opportunities to talk to other people. Try new activities, such as crafts, sports, speaking groups, and socialize with people after the activity. Develop conversational skills by talking about different topics. Take an interest in other people – do not wait for them to get interested in you first. If you find yourself avoiding a situation, you should begin by tackling a similar but slightly easier situation and then work your way up to trying the harder one again once you have increased your confidence at the lower level. Do the following:

140

- practice your social skills with others in relaxed situations;
- consider how people act towards you and all the different interpretations you can put on their behaviour – they may be reacting to you in a particular way for reasons other than your stammer;
- look on a social situation as an opportunity for you to experiment with a new skill or strategy or to continue to develop an old one;
- try to think of problematical social situations as something to learn from and build upon, and remember to balance these with your successes;
- think of negative reactions as the other person's problem, not yours.

You as your own clinician

- Review the notes you made and/or the objectives and targets you set in therapy from time to time.
- Explain your therapy to your family, friends, colleagues and so on and enlist their help in keeping you working at your speech. Have them experiment with one or two of the techniques just for fun!
- Keep your toolbox with you at all times and allocate one time slot every day when you can read it over to yourself.
- Try to maintain an analytical approach to your speech and use problem-solving techniques when necessary.
- Balance the good times with the not-so-good times.
- Be kind to yourself. Take care of your diet, sleeping pattern, nutrition and so on. Reward yourself for working hard, taking risks, trying something new. You deserve it!

11
Concluding remarks

So, we come to the end of this book. We hope it has been useful to you. If you stammer, we hope it has given you belief in yourself, that you can change in some way, be it the intensity of your actual stammering, your communication skills or the way you feel about speaking and about yourself. If you do not stammer but have read the book because you know someone who does, our wish is that you now understand a little more about this complicated area and why so much patience, courage and motivation are needed to bring about change. Perhaps this understanding can make it easier for you to offer support and encouragement in that change and a shoulder to cry on in those times when the person you know finds the struggle too great.

At the Oxford Dysfluency Conference in June 1996, one speaker, Dodo Astrup, referred to stammering as a 'sore spot'. She described this as the vulnerable part of a person which has been carefully hidden for so many years. When the person decides the time has come to change, they have to expose this sore spot, to take away the sticking plaster, bandages and all that has protected them from being hurt. We were describing this to one of our clients and she felt it made a great deal of sense. She described the process rather more graphically, telling us it was rather like someone asking us to expose our bottoms to the world and show every bit of cellulite to all and sundry!

Yes, confronting stammering is hard. However, it can also be immensely rewarding and freeing, like unlocking a prisoner's door, taking off their shackles and letting them breathe the fresh air. If you stammer, we want to encourage you to escape from the prison of stammering and to let yourself and others see the real you. A word of warning, though – don't rush at the changes; take it gradually. Go on parole first! Try out new ways of being and behaving slowly, one step at a time. Allow yourself to get it wrong sometimes, to make mistakes, revert to old behaviours. It's all part of learning. In these difficult times, you are likely to need support from those close to you. Ask for it! Talking over your difficulties can help you get them into perspective, to unload some of that heavy burden you have been carrying and begin to get yourself back on the right track.

We wish you well in your journey of discovery.

142

Appendix I: easy onset word practice lists

Vowels

arm	ear	in	one	use
ant	easy	is	only	unite
ass	early	issue	oven	under
ally	energy	illness	often	useful
after	elbow	immense	ordinary	umbrella

Easy consonants

have	love	man	noon	five	run
hello	lady	mill	name	feet	ruin
halo	late	move	nice	favour	realize
hush	luck	much	need	foolish	rift
happy	lift	mountain	night	fix	rat

sun	view	will	you
say	vase	wave	young
sell	vile	west	yellow
soft	village	weak	yacht
sink	vex	wonder	yeast

Harder consonants

boy	cat	dry	good	June	pat
beetle	cry	dish	gift	July	pie
buy	cuddle	day	game	jolly	pull
baby	cost	dark	got	just	pin
belt	cool	deep	go	jif	post

try
tie
tan
tooth
tuck

APPENDIX 1: EASY ONSET WORD PRACTICE LISTS

Two-word phrases

any route	very valuable	nice outfit
easy action	which way	rosy cheeks
inner harmony	silly sausage	perfect picture
open house	young saver	blue sky
under floor	many roads	daft prank
great day	lazy lad	cute kitten
try harder		

Short phrases

How many people where there?	Many a slip twixt cup and lip.	Try to get one.
When are you coming?	Nearly but not quite.	Don't forget to go.
Are there many of them?	You must be joking.	Cut it up very small.
Easy come, easy go?	Go to the end of the road.	Half a box of mushrooms.
Out of sight, out of mind.	Will she, won't she?	Just the two of us.
It's an ill wind.	See how they run.	Listen to me.
Up and down the hill.	Vacuum the stairs.	Quiet in there please!
She sells seashells.	Buy me some bread.	Take me to Ted.
Fill up your glass.	Put the kettle on.	
Run and get them.		

Appendix II: a relaxation routine

Do this at a time when you will not be interrupted and are not so tired that you are likely to fall asleep. You will need about 15 minutes.

Although you are relaxing, you will also need to concentrate hard on what you are doing. Start this routine off by sitting in a chair or lying on the bed. Loosen your clothing so you do not feel restricted. Relax your body in a way similar to the one we outline below. You may find it helpful to start by asking someone to read out the text that follows slowly, or you could read it yourself onto a tape which you could then play back.

Start off by thinking about your breathing. Notice the slow, steady rhythm. Think about breathing in and breathing out. As you breathe in, feel yourself breathing in a feeling of calm and relaxation. As you breathe out, imagine the tension leaving your body through your mouth and the tips of your fingers and toes. Take a minute or two to just concentrate on your breathing and on feeling the relaxation start to spread through your body.

Now think about your hands and arms. Notice where your hands make contact with the chair or bed. Become aware of the temperature of the skin of your hands – their warmth or coolness. Notice any tingling sensations in the ends of your fingers. As you become aware of the tension, it begins to go and is replaced by relaxation. Tension replaced by relaxation.

Think about your arms and the position of your arms on the chair or bed. Notice any tension in your arms, across your shoulders and all across your neck and back. As you become aware of the tension, it begins to go and is replaced by relaxation. Tension replaced by relaxation.

Now think of your feet and legs. Be aware of the warmth or coolness of the skin of your feet. Notice any tingling sensations in the ends of your toes. As you become aware of the tension, it begins to go and is replaced by relaxation. Tension replaced by relaxation. Now think of your legs and notice where the back of your legs rest on the chair or the bed. Be aware of any tension in the muscles of your legs, and as you become aware of the tension, it begins to go and is replaced by relaxation. Tension replaced by relaxation.

Your hands, arms, feet and legs are now becoming heavy and relaxed. Feel yourself sinking back now into the chair or bed as you become even more relaxed.

Think now of the muscles of your face, first of all around your forehead and eyes. Become aware of any frowning tension there. Now notice around your mouth and jaws and become aware of any clenching tension there. Be

145

aware of the position of your tongue in your mouth. Are you pushing it against your teeth or your palate? As you notice the tension, it begins to go and is replaced by relaxation. Tension replaced by relaxation.

Your whole body is now feeling relaxed. Continue holding on to this feeling of relaxation by imagining a scene which you associate with calm and relaxation. It may be a scene you know or it could be an imaginary one – a countryside or seaside scene or anything else you choose. Spend some time in your scene and let its peace and calmness help you feel even more relaxed. Notice any remaining pockets of tension and then let them go.

When you feel ready, finish off the relaxation routine by counting back from six to one, gradually becoming less heavy as you do so, but still keeping that feeling of relaxation. Take time to open your eyes and make sure you have a good stretch. Take your time getting up from the bed or chair.

Further reading

Alberti, R., and Emmons, M., *Your Perfect Right: A guide to assertive living*, Penguin Books, New York, 1981

Back, K., and Back, K., *Assertiveness at Work* McGraw-Hill Book Company, 1992

Breitenfeldt, D. H., and Lorenz, D. R., *Successful Stuttering Management Program*, Eastern Washington University, Cheney, Washington, 1989

British Association for Counselling (BAC), 'Counselling and Psychotherapy: Is it for me? (leaflet, 4th edition), available from BAC, 1994

Cutman, J. *The Assertiveness Workbook: A plan for busy women* Sheldon Press, 1993

Eaglen, Diane, and Plummer, Debs, *You Can Change: A self-help guide to the management of stress*, available from Speech and Language Therapy Department, Fosse Health Trust, Yeoman House, 5a Yeoman Street, Leicester LE1 1US, tel. 01533 516811

Fransella, F., *Personal Change and Reconstruction*, Academic Press, 1972

Hauck, P. *How to Stand up for Yourself*, Sheldon Press, 1981

Holland, S., and Ward, C., *Assertiveness: A practical approach*, Winslow Press, 1990

Hunt, B., 'Self-help for stutterers – experience in Britain', in Rustin, L., Purser, H., and Rowley, D. (Eds), *Progress in the Treatment of Fluency Disorders*, Taylor and Francis, 1987

Kelly, G. A., *The Psychology of Personal Constructs*, Routledge, 1991

Lindenfield, G., *Assert Yourself: How to reprogramme your mind for positive action*, Thorsons, 1987

McKay, M., Davis, M., and Fanning, P., *Messages: The communication skills workbook*, New Harbinger, Oakland, C.A., 1983

Pease, A., *Body Language: How to read others' thoughts by their gestures*, Sheldon Press, 1984

Prochaska, J. O., Norcross, J. C., and DiClemente, C. C., *Changing for Good*, William Morrow & Co. Inc., New York, 1994

Scheffer, Mechthild, *Bach Flower Therapy*, Thorsons, 1996

Sheehan, J. G., 'Conflict Theory and Avoidance-reduction Therapy' in Eisenson, J. (Ed.), *Stuttering: A second symposium*, Harper & Row, New York, 1975

Smith, M. T., *When I Say No I Feel Guilty*, Bantam Books, New York, 1975

Snaith, R. P., 'A method of psychotherapy based on relaxation techniques', *British Journal of Psychiatry*, 124, pp. 473–81, 1974

Turnbull, J., and Stewart, T., *Helping Children Cope with Stammering*, Sheldon Press, 1996

Waxman, D., *Hartland's Medical and Dental Hypnosis* (3rd Edition), Unwin Paperbacks, 1989

Scientific journals

European Journal of Disorders of Communication
Journal of Fluency Disorders
Journal of Speech and Hearing Disorders
Journal of Speech and Hearing Research

Useful addresses

British Stammering Association
15 Old Ford Road
Bethnal Green
London E2 9PJ
Tel: 0181 983 1003

British Association for Counselling
1 Regent Place
Rugby
Warwickshire CV21 2PJ
Tel: 01788 578328/550899

Royal College of Speech and Language Therapists
7 Bath Place
Rivington Street
London EC2A 3DR
Tel. 0171 613 3855

Index